Dr Newton trained at King's College Hospital, London and then completed a general practice vocational training scheme in Humberside. Following this experience in family practice he moved back into hospital general paediatrics and developed a specific interest in child and adolescent neurology. Following higher specialist training he was appointed as Consultant Paediatric Neurologist to the Children's Hospitals in Manchester in 1983, where he was Director of Clerical Services, latterly Medical Director from 1988–98. From 2001 to 2004 he was President of the British Paediatric Neurology Association. His doctoral thesis was written on aspects of the scope for intervention in pregnancy to prevent low birthweight and reduce the incidence of cerebral palsy. He has a son with Down's syndrome and has been a member of the Down's Syndrome Association since 1985.

The Down's Syndrome Handbook

A practical guide for parents and carers

Dr Richard Newton
MD FRCPCH FRCP MRCGP DCH DRCOG

Written in conjunction with the Down's Syndrome Association

Illustrated by
Jennie Smith

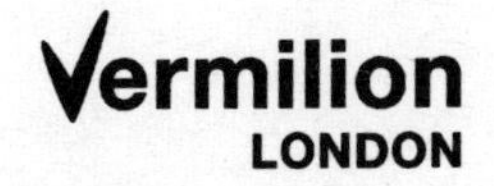

3 5 7 9 10 8 6 4

First published in the United Kingdom by Optima in 1992

First published in the United Kingdom by Vermilion in 1997

This revised edition published in the United Kingdom in 2004 by Vermilion, an imprint of Ebury Press
Random House UK Ltd
Random House
20 Vauxhall Bridge Road
London SW1V 2SA

Random House Australia (Pty) Limited
20 Alfred Street, Milsons Point, Sydney,
New South Wales 2061, Australia

Random House New Zealand Limited
18 Poland Road, Glenfield,
Auckland 10, New Zealand

Random House (Pty) Limited
Endulini, 5A Jubilee Road, Parktown 2193, South Africa

Random House UK Limited Reg. No. 954009
www.randomhouse.co.uk
Papers used by Vermilion are natural, recyclable products made from wood grown in sustainable forests.

A CIP catalogue record is available for this book from the British Library.

ISBN: 0091884306

Typeset by Deltatype Limited, Birkenhead, Merseyside

Printed and bound in Great Britain by
Mackays of Chatham plc, Chatham, Kent

CONTENTS

To Judith, Sarah, Michael and Jennifer
as part payment for the time I should have spent
with them whilst writing this text.
***And** to the*
DOWN'S SYNDROME ASSOCIATION
for their continuing help and encouragement of
PEOPLE WITH SPECIAL NEEDS

ACKNOWLEDGEMENTS

A number of people need appreciative thanks for their contribution to this work. The original project was the idea of Sue Brooks, past-director of the Down's Syndrome Association, and she made a major contribution to the first edition text, along with Elizabeth Blackwell of the South East branch of the DSA, Shirley Quemby and Jean Shergold.

For the new edition special thanks are due to Carol Boys, DSA Chief Executive, and Susannah Seyman, Information Officer, for tireless effort in helping to bring the whole thing together. Bob Black, DSA Education Information Officer, Sally Capper, Education Advocacy Worker, and Christina Katic, DSA Welfare Benefits Advisor, helped with extensive updating of the relevant sections. The photographs are from the DSA Photo Library.

Special thanks are due to Zaid Sheehan for updating the section on hearing and the ear, nose and throat.

I am most grateful to Margaret Cunnah for her continuing help and the original typing of the manuscript.

Finally, I should like to thank Cliff Cunningham and his team, and scientists everywhere who through painstaking work have helped establish the facts about Down's syndrome and dispense with the unhelpful myths.

PREFACE

This book has been written to complement existing introductory texts on Down's syndrome, by exploring in more detail many of the common questions raised by parents. In so doing it will clearly be of use not only to parents, family members, teachers and social workers, but also to doctors, health workers and medical students.

Our intention is not to provide an exhaustive supply of specialised information but rather to provide up-to-date general information and, more importantly, practical help and advice. It is hoped that this will assist each person in their attempt to provide encouragement and opportunity for babies, children and adults with Down's syndrome to flourish and reach their full potential.

The majority of people who read this book may only have the opportunity to encounter a small number of people with Down's syndrome. It is the aim of this book to help them make the most of that opportunity.

1

Introduction

> 'If I could do it then anyone could.' The words of Peter Wiseman, aged 35, having completed his first parachute jump; nothing particularly remarkable about this perhaps, except that Peter has Down's syndrome.
>
> 'I would like to be called by my name, not by what's wrong with me.' A plea from Anya Souza, who also has Down's syndrome, and who, once employed at the national office of the Down's Syndrome Association, is now pursuing a career as a freelance artist.

Two exceptional people who have one thing in common, namely a genetic condition known as Down's syndrome. However, there the similarity ends. Peter and Anya come from very different backgrounds and upbringing, but both have developed a determination not to be typecast by others as a result of their outward appearance or by the label of this particular form of learning disability. Compared with many children and adults with Down's syndrome, Peter and Anya are high achievers. This has come about through hard work and the support and encouragement of families and enlightened professionals. They have set an example which many could follow. We now live in a world that offers people with Down's syndrome more opportunity than ever before. This introduction will briefly explore how it is we came to be where we are today.

Down's syndrome is not a disease; it is a genetic condition affecting 800 to 1,000 live births each year in the UK. Children and adults with Down's syndrome are not sufferers or victims; they happen to share some physical characteristics, and also have a degree of learning disability, which varies from person to person. It is important always to remember that however similar babies and children may look at first glance, they carry family likenesses that become obvious quite quickly. It is also important to remember that physical characteristics are no indication of future ability or capacity to learn.

Attitudes to people with Down's syndrome have changed over the years, but many of the old prejudices and myths remain. In the rural communities of an earlier age such differences were manageable, but as times changed so did people's attitudes, and little differentiation was made between people who were 'mad', merely 'different' in some way, or just plain 'bad'. The inmates at Bedlam – the Bethlehem Royal Hospital, and the first asylum for the insane in England – and other asylums, were put on show as curiosities. Those with less extreme forms of visible difference were locked away in large institutions, often in the most beautiful country settings, to save them from doing harm to themselves or to others. With very few other resources and little knowledge about their potential, people were cared for, to a greater or lesser degree, for many years, miles away from their home and community.

People with Down's syndrome were no exception to this general attitude, but it was not until the middle of the last century that Dr Langdon Down first identified a group of people in an institution and gave the collection of characteristics he had observed an identity. At this time the Victorian medical world had discovered the science of classification. Dr Down, working with the scientific beliefs of the era, concluded that this group of people was a sub-species of the human race, a throwback to 'inferior' non-European races.

Down coined the term 'Mongolian idiots'; variations he called 'negroid idiots', 'Aztec idiots' and 'Malaysian idiots', but none of these latter terms entered the language. Unfortunately, the term 'mongol' became an entrenched part of our language, conjuring up an image of institutional care.

Thankfully, the term Mongol is no longer in use today. It was replaced largely in the early 1990s by 'people with Down's syndrome'. People, even occasionally professionals, will be heard to say 'Down's syndrome people', or 'Down's syndrome children' – the important point is that they are *people* first, and 'people with Down's syndrome' is better.

People with Down's syndrome, of course, just regard themselves as people and one day it is to be hoped this is the way we all shall think. In the words of the Down's Syndrome Association promotional campaign they are 'people with prospects'. The main difference between a person with Down's syndrome and an average person in the population is that we are beginning to know how the former's genetic make-up may determine their strengths and weaknesses. With the current rate of advance of genetic knowledge, that may apply to us all before too long!

It was in the 1950s that Professor Jerome Lejeune, working in Paris, discovered that the features that made Down's syndrome so distinctive were genetic in origin. In discovering that an extra chromosome was the cause of Down's syndrome he started a process of understanding that continues to advance day by day. We now know exactly which part of chromosome 21 leads to the distinctive features of Down's syndrome. We now even know the relatively short sequence of genes on chromosome 21 involved, which protein the genes produce and how the function of cells in the body may be affected. Clearly, one day this knowledge may lead us to be able to lessen the effect of the over-active genes, but for the moment this seems to be a long way off.

Alongside the significant advances in scientific knowledge have been significant changes in education. Most children with Down's syndrome now should have the opportunity to be integrated into mainstream education, with appropriate support; their secondary education in many Authorities is also linked to employment opportunity. Many people with Down's syndrome are now able to lead at least a semi-independent existence in the community, and follow college courses according to their level of ability. Society is becoming aware that a learning impairment may not after all be such a disadvantage if appropriate opportunities and encouragement are offered.

2

What is Down's syndrome?

In 1866 Langdon Down first described the characteristics of the commonest recognisable cause of learning disability in Britain. In 1959, 93 years later, Lejeune showed that Down's syndrome was due to extra genetic material carried on chromosome 21, and since that time it has been shown that the characteristics of Down's syndrome are related to a relatively small part of the long arm of chromosome 21, (21q22.1–21q22.3).

This section of the chromosome carries perhaps only 50 to 100 genes. This is a small proportion of the total of the 30,000 genes to be found on the whole of human genome (see below).

Since 1866, theories on the causation of Down's syndrome and the mechanism of brain impairment have altered radically. In the 19th century, when Down was alive, it was thought that the foetus went through developmental stages in which it assumed different racial characteristics. The legacy of the theory persisted, and as recently as 1978 a book was published with the sub-title *The Psychology of Mongolism*. In the same year as Lejeune identified trisomy 21, a paper appeared relating the incidence of Down's syndrome to increased levels of stress in pregnancy. Now Down's syndrome has replaced the term Mongolism in scientific literature, and better understanding has allowed us to dispense with spurious beliefs about causation.

It is still not fully known what predisposes dividing cells to retain extra chromosomal material, how this extra material disrupts normal development, nor how function is disrupted as a result. This chapter will summarise the current state of knowledge on these issues and serve to emphasise how much there is yet to be known.

Human genetics

First it is useful to outline some of the basic facts about human genetics.

One of the most exciting developments of the 20th century was the identification of DNA (deoxyribonucleic acid) as one of the secrets of life itself. DNA is composed of nucleic acids linked with sugars capable of forming very long chains and has the further very important property of being able to reproduce and replicate itself. It appears in human cells as a double-stranded helix (spiral); two strands of the spiralled ladder being connected by struts of chemicals called purines and pyrimidines. The two purines involved are called adenine and thymidine, whilst the two pyrimidines are known as cytosine and guanine. The sequence of these basepairs on the DNA molecule is very important in governing cell activity, for it is this sequence that gives the instructing code for which proteins are going to be produced within the cell. Some sections on the DNA molecule code for proteins involved in the structure of the cell; other sections code for proteins known as enzymes, which regulate the activity of chemical reactions within the cell. Any disruption of the structure of DNA would clearly lead to a disruption of either cell structure or cell function, or both.

Most DNA within a human cell is concentrated in the cell nucleus, which looks denser under the microscope than the rest of the cell contents. Within the cell nucleus the DNA strands are divided up into very small structures called chromosomes. In humans there are 23 pairs of chromosomes, 22 of which are identical, while the 23rd pair (referred to as an X or Y chromosome) determines the sex of an individual. The chromosomes vary in size. The larger chromosomes carry more genes and therefore govern more activity within the cell than the smaller ones.

Each chromosome is made up of two strands of DNA, each referred to as a chromatid. The chromatids are joined together by chiasmata, which are strands of non-genetic material. Along part of the length of the chromosome the chromatids are very obviously joined together at a specific site known as the centromere. This is usually not in the centre, which means that each chromatid has a long arm and a short arm. The short arm of a chromosome is referred to as p, whilst the long arm is referred to as q. With the special staining technique known as banding, the chromosomes can be divided up into segments. Smaller segments on the DNA molecule which code for

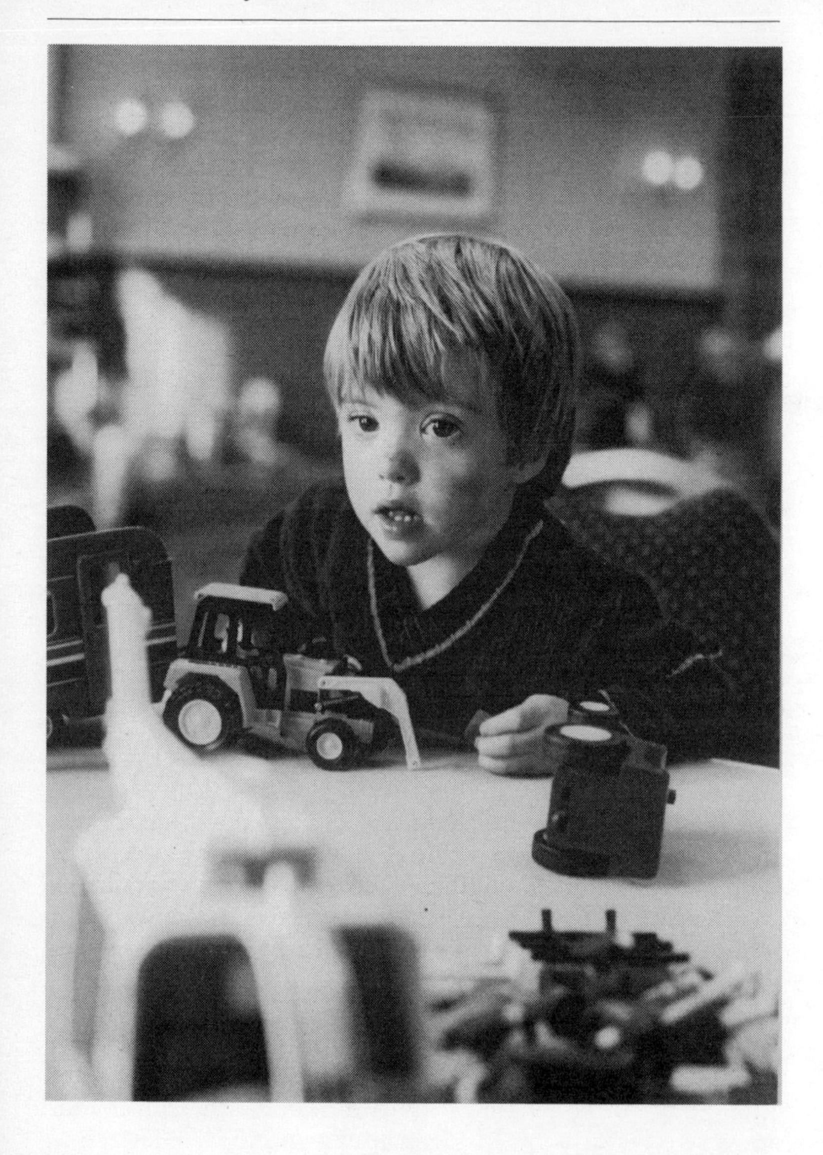

Down's syndrome is not a disease; it is a genetic condition. Children with Down's syndrome are not sufferers or victims; they are people with special, additional needs.

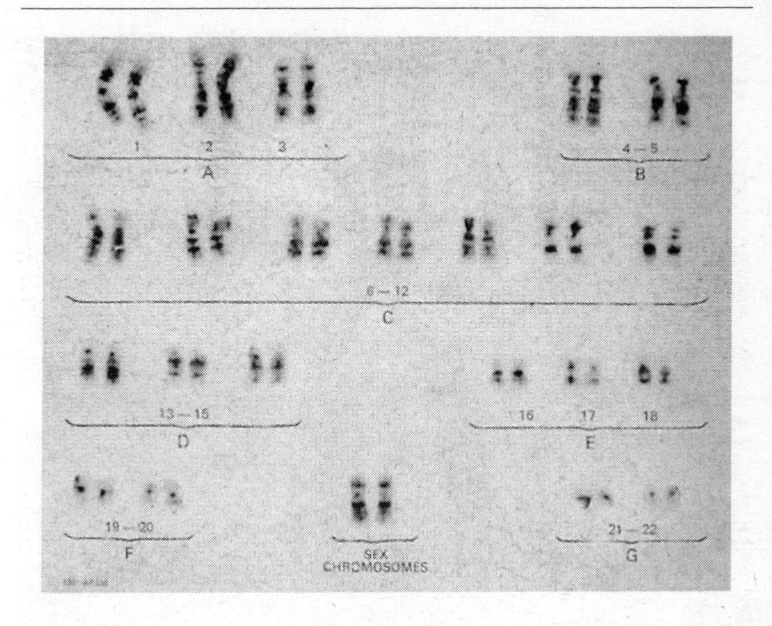

Human chromosomes from a normal female cell – 23 pairs and two X (female) chromosomes.

particular proteins are known as genes. The extra chromosomal material that leads to the features of Down's syndrome is found on chromosome 21, between segments 21q22.1 and 22.3. This means that the chromosomal material is found between the first and third parts of the 22nd segment on the long arm of chromosome 21. This small portion of the whole human genome accounts for perhaps only 50 to 100 genes, the function of only a few of which has been identified to date.

Cell division

Somatic division or mitosis

Cells in every tissue in the body are constantly being produced and then die off. This production of cells involves an individual cell line dividing and then dividing again to

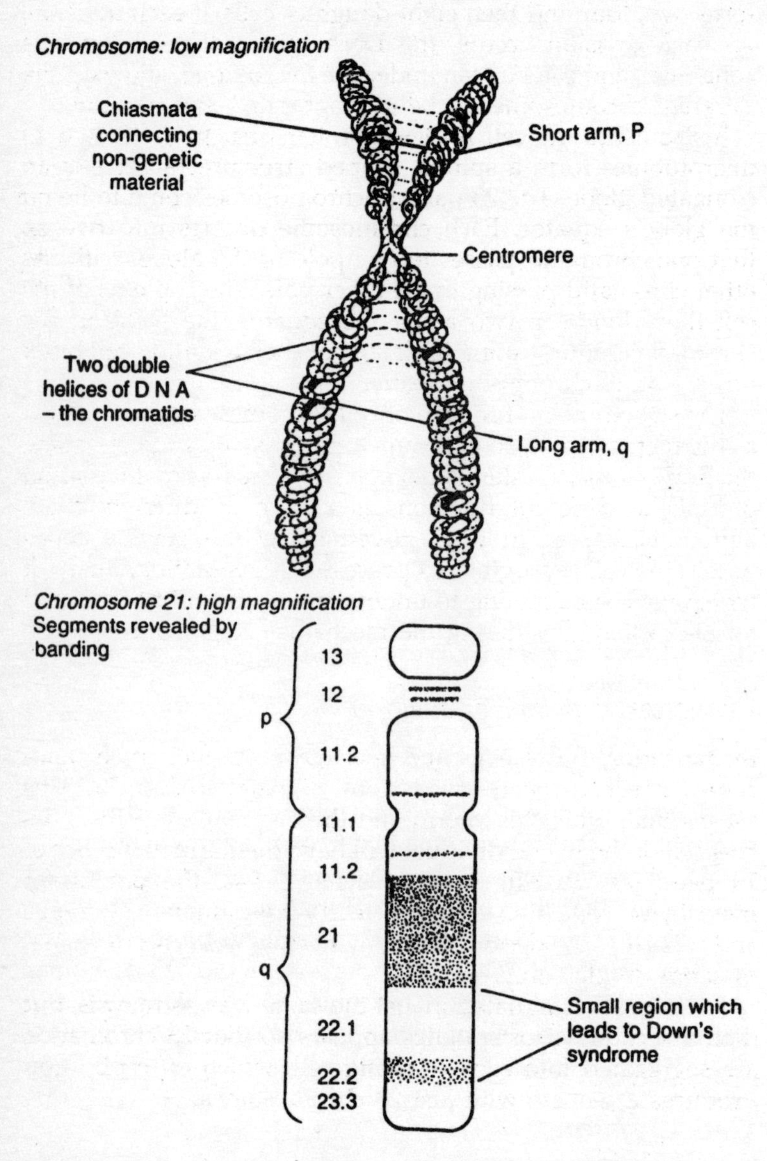

Diagram of chromosome 21 at high magnification. The different segments are revealed by a technique known as banding.

form two, four and then eight daughter cells at each division. As each division occurs, the DNA within the cell nucleus condenses and can be seen under the microscope, allowing the different chromosomes to be photographed and identified.

Just outside the cell nucleus, protein structures known as microtubules form a spindle-shaped structure rather like an elongated globe. The 23 pairs of chromosomes come to lie on the globe's equator. Each chromosome divides into two so that one chromatid passes to one pole of the globe, with the other chromatid passing to the other pole. The contents of the cell then divide in two along the equator, the DNA in the chromatids reduplicating itself so that each resulting cell has a full set of 23 chromosome pairs.

The structure and function of cells becomes very specialised as the foetus grows, so that some cells make up muscles, some the brain, some the skin and so on. This process of adaptation of cells to different functions is known as differentiation. Differentiation is, in turn, governed by the genetic codes within the cell through strict processes of regulation, many of which we are beginning to understand. This will be returned to later when considering the mechanism of impairment.

Reduction division or meiosis

In the formation of eggs and sperm the number of chromosomes needs to be reduced from 23 pairs to just 23. This means that, when the sperm and the egg come together, the first cell of the new individual will have the normal number of 23 pairs restored. In order to achieve this, the process of meiosis, or reduction division, leads the gamete cells (eggs and sperm) to divide twice, whereas the chromosomal material divides only once.

The process is initiated in just the same way as mitosis, but then a second set of spindles appears so that 23 chromatids are segregated into each resulting cell, which on replication produces a gamete with just 23 chromosomes.

Disordered division

- *Non-disjunction.* If a cell divides and more chromosomal material goes to one pole than the other, then the daughter cells produced will have an abnormal number of chromo-

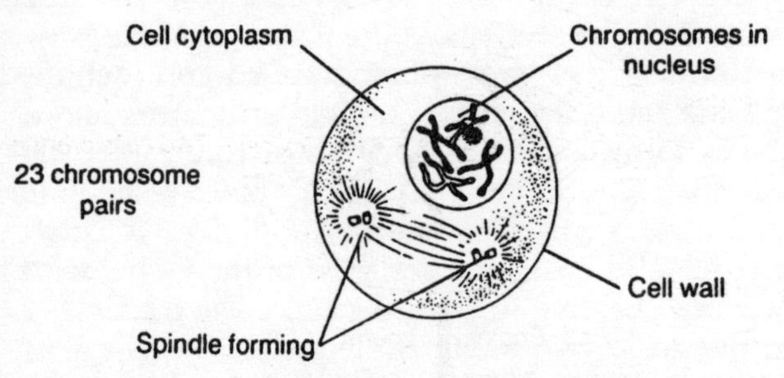

Chromosomes become visible in nucleus. Spindle begins to form.

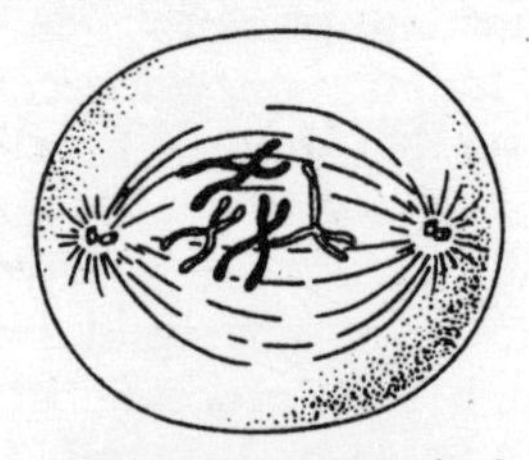

Nucleus wall breaks up, chromosomes attached to spindle by centromere.

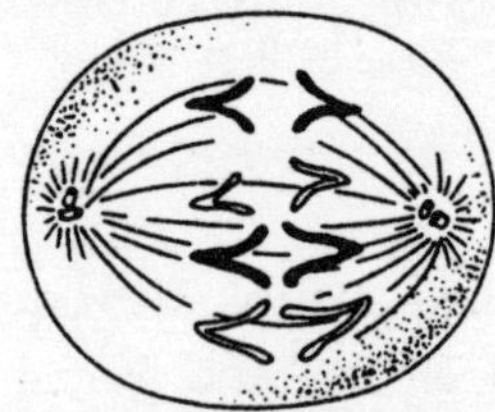

Each chromosome splits in two – one chromatid to one pole and one to the other.

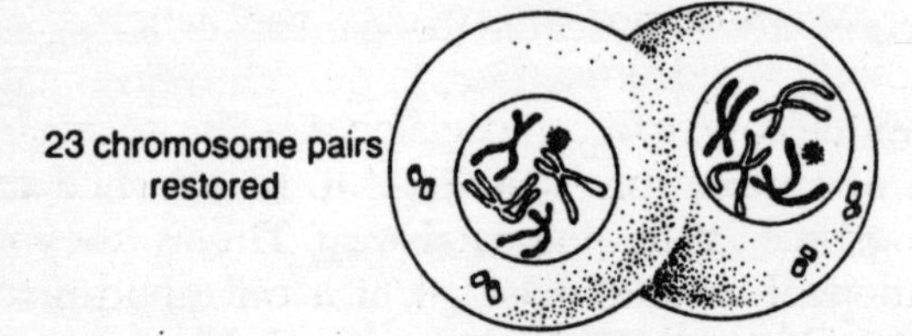

The D N A replicates – each chromatid becomes a new daughter chromosome. A nucleus wall reforms and the cytoplasm splits to give the complete daughter cells.

The sequence of events in mitosis – somatic division.

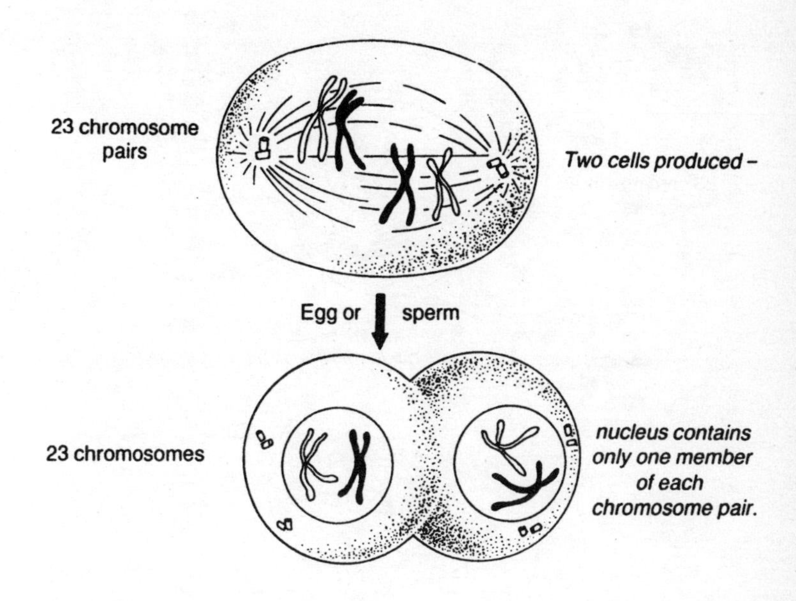

Formation of egg and sperm. The first meiotic or reduction division.

somes. This is called aneuploidy; one will show too many chromosomes (hyperploidy) and one too few (hypoploidy). This disordered movement of chromosomes is called non-disjunction and is the commonest cause of the trisomy (three chromosomes rather than the usual pair) that causes Down's syndrome.

- *Translocation.* In the course of cell division it is also possible for a segment of chromosomal material to be attached to another chromosome in an abnormal way. This is known as a translocation of genetic material. If a cell divides to produce a daughter cell with the normal 23 pairs of chromosomes plus a translocation of material from chromosome 21, this will lead to the features of Down's syndrome. On the other hand it is possible, depending on how the chromosomes segregate on the equator of the spindle at cell division, for the translocated material to go to the same pole of the spindle as the chromosome from

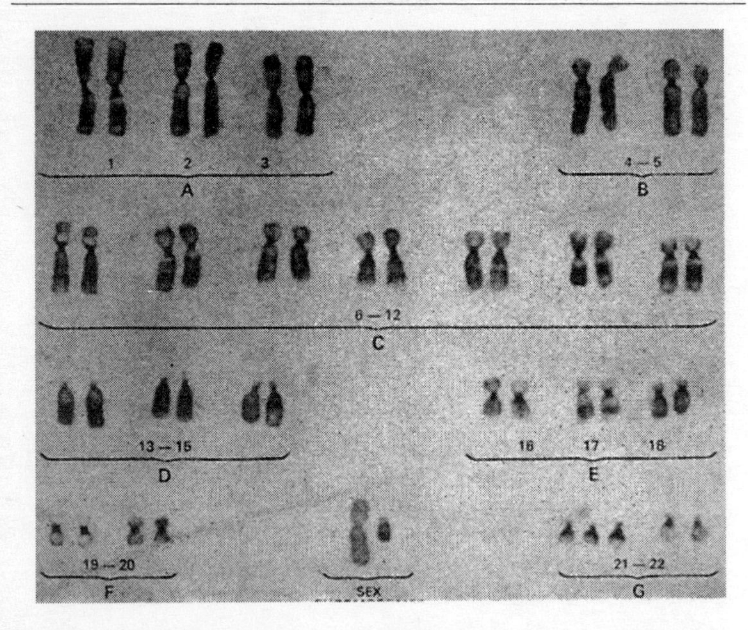

Human chromosomes, showing trisomy 21. Note the three chromosomes at the 21 position, instead of the usual two.

which this extra material broke off. In these circumstances one chromosome would be smaller than usual whilst another would carry the extra genetic material. This is known as a balanced translocation and the person is likely to be normal.

- *Mosaicism.* If cell division goes wrong at the stage of early foetal development, but after the first few somatic divisions, then only a few cell lines may be involved in translocation or non-disjunction. In this case examination of different tissues of the body will show that some cells have the normal number of chromosomes whereas others show extra genetic material. This is known as mosaicism.

Disordered division and Down's syndrome

If a person carries the extra segment of chromosomal material from chromosome 21 (segments 21q22.1–21q22.3) they will

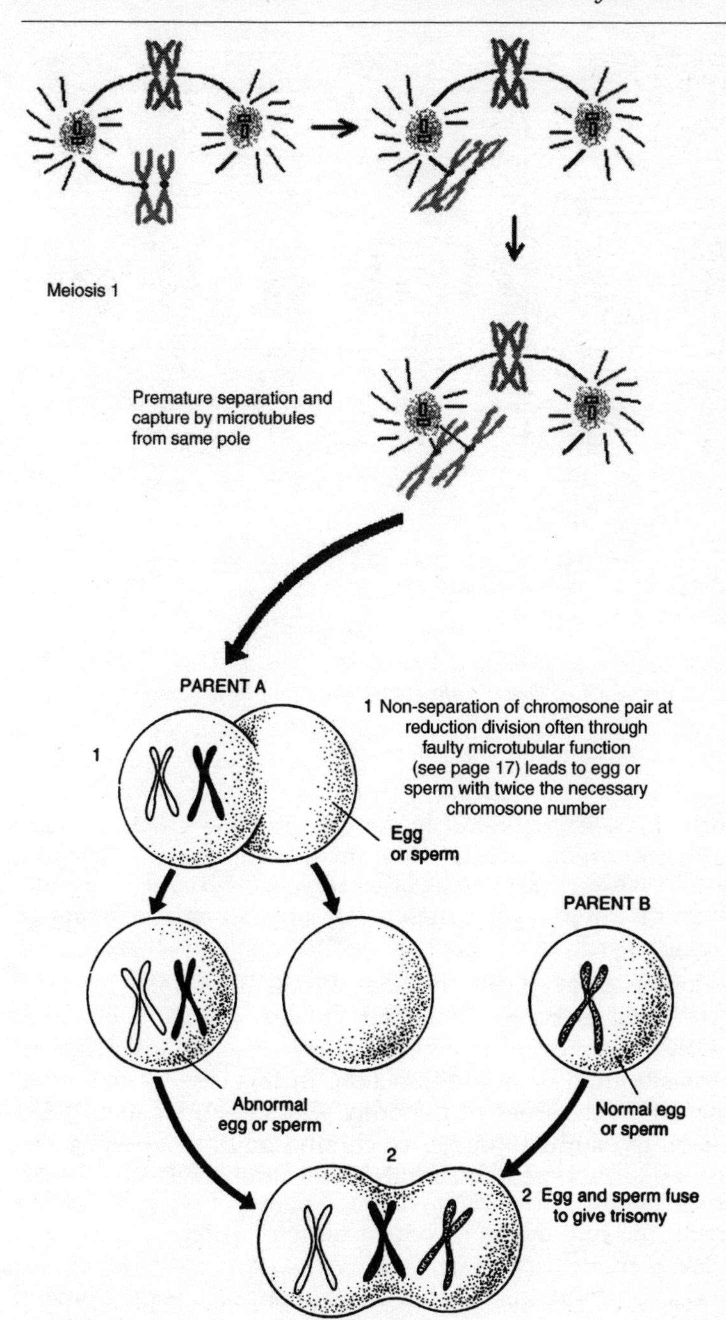

Diagrammatic representation of non-disjunction.

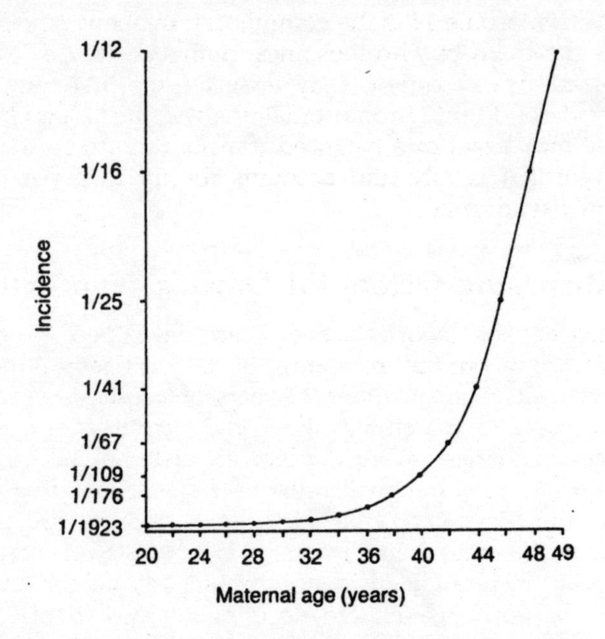

Incidence of Down's syndrome according to maternal age.

have Down's syndrome, whether it be through a non-disjunction of the chromosomal material or a translocation. The range of abilities therefore is likely to be the same in each group. For people with mosaicism, however, relatively few cell lines can be affected and on the whole this group tend to have relatively less disability. It must be said, however, that there is a huge overlap in the ability of people with Down's syndrome mosaicism and those with other forms of Down's syndrome.

Down's syndrome is most commonly due to trisomy 21. The trisomy arises because of a non-disjunction of chromosomes at the reduction division. Trisomy may arise either during the first or the second meiotic division.

About 5 per cent of children with Down's syndrome will have a translocation, the extra chromosome 21 material having attached itself to one of the D group (chromosomes 13, 14 or

15). Chromosome 14 is the commonest. In about 1 per cent of cases the G group chromosomes, numbers 21 or 22, will be involved. Translocations may arise for the first time in the affected child, but chromosomal analysis in the parents may reveal mosaicism or a balanced translocation to be the cause.

Mosaicism is rare and accounts for up to 5 per cent of Down's syndrome.

Predisposing factors for Down's syndrome

A number of theories have been developed to explain observations on the incidence of Down's syndrome. The incidence in women under 20 years of age is less than 1 in 2,000, rising to something like 1 in 20 at the age of 45. The steepest increment in incidence with maternal age occurs at the age of 35, although it must be remembered that half of those mothers who give birth to a child with Down's syndrome are less than 35 years old. In recent years there has been an increasing incidence amongst younger mothers, partly because women are deciding to have their families earlier.

There are clearly factors other than maternal age that are important, increasing paternal age being one of these.

The effect of paternal age on incidence of Down's syndrome

Paternal age	*Maternal age*	
	35–40 (%)	41–46 (%)
34	0.4	0.8
35–40	0.6	1.2
41–46	1.3	2.8
47	2.0	4.1

After Stene *et al.*, 1981.

Although the impact of paternal age is not as marked as that of maternal age, the effect seems to be derived from the ageing of sperm. Animal studies have shown that the longer sperm is stored in the genito-urinary tract, the greater the incidence there is of sperm-derived trisomies. Decreased frequency of sexual intercourse means that the sperm ejaculated are relatively older. Until recently, it was thought that this could be part of the explanation for the higher incidence of Down's syndrome in babies born to older couples, who might have had a decreased frequency of sexual intercourse. It was also considered as a possible explanation for the increasing number of babies with Down's syndrome born to unmarried teenage couples who, because they did not live together, did not have intercourse as frequently as co-habiting/married couples. However, recent studies have suggested that this is unlikely to be the explanation, in either group.

It is possible to determine the parental origin of the extra chromosomal material by studying chromosomal variants (heteromorphisms). A number of studies have reliably shown that in about 80 per cent of trisomies the extra chromosome has its origins in non-disjunction at the first maternal reduction division. There is then no support for the theory that the 'older' eggs of an 'older woman' increase the risk of trisomy; this first meiosis takes place in the ovary long before the mother herself is born.

The remainder of heteromorphisms take their origin in the second maternal meiotic division or in the first or second paternal meiotic divisions. It is known that the crossover of chromosomal material and non-disjunction may be caused by reduced chiasmata formation, the chiasmata being the non-genetic strands that help paired chromosomes adhere to each other. Chiasmata formation occurs before birth in females and reduces with age, making it more likely for genetic material to split off in an abnormal way. Increasing maternal age therefore leads to an increase in the number of cells with an abnormal number of chromosomes.

The development of many abnormal embryos is arrested by a process called micronucleation or extrusion of nuclei which carry an abnormal number of chromosomes (aneuploidy). Thus the vast majority of pregnancies involving abnormal foetuses miscarry spontaneously, often at a very early stage. Research is currently focusing on whether the increased production of abnormal embryos is the sole cause of the increased frequency with age, or whether there is actually a decrease in this natural process of selective destruction.

Foetuses showing a reduced number of chromosomes

(hypoploidy) cannot survive, as the effect on the growing metabolism is too great. Hyperploidy (too many) of the larger chromosomes, with their great effect on body metabolism, also seems to lead to foetal death. However, hyperploidy of the smaller chromosomes, with a lesser effect, is often compatible with survival. As chromosome 21 is one of the smallest, Down's syndrome comes to be the commonest recognisable form of learning disability.

The development of more sophisticated techniques has led to greater insights into the ways in which the reduction division may go wrong. One of these techniques, using DNA probes that recognise specific points on the chromosome, has allowed scientists to map out chromosome 21 and define the point of any chromosomal abnormality. To date, 50 such markers are available, allowing up to 100 per cent accuracy in the prediction of the site and type of abnormality. This technique will doubtlessly improve our future understanding.

The part that environmental factors, such as X-rays, chemicals and viruses, may play on some of these chromosomal events is as yet undefined. Hormonal factors may be of importance; an increased frequency of chromosome abnormality has been noted in the pregnancies that miscarry in women of any age who are users of the contraceptive pill. It can readily be seen how male workers in areas of radiation exposure may suffer abnormalities at the first and second paternal meiotic division, as the production of new sperm goes on throughout life.

There also may be inherent biological vulnerability factors in some individuals, outside environmental influence. For example one study showed the cells of mothers of children with Down's syndrome to have a variation of microtubular function. The microtubules form the spindle on which the separation of the chromosomes takes place at the time of cell division. Studies have shown that this 'conveyor belt' function becomes inefficient with age. Premature separation and capture of both pairs of like chromosomes at the first meiotic division (see page 13) leads to the trisomy.

Prevention

At present there seems to be little scope for prevention in Down's syndrome. The environmental factors cited above have no more than speculative importance at this stage, although if any were to become better defined, attention to safety standards at work and political influences of an environmental and ecological nature could lead to a reduction in background risk.

Further study may help us identify those with a genetic predisposition, and appropriate counselling could ensue.

Characteristics of Down's syndrome

The phenotype refers to the observable features of a genetic condition; it includes physical appearance, behaviour and intellectual function.

Down's syndrome – phenotype

Hypotonia – flexible joints
Learning difficulties
Mild microcephaly – brachycephaly
Epicanthic folds – Mongoloid slant – Brushfield spots
Lens opacity – refractive error
Small ears
Dentition – hypoplasia, irregular placement
– less caries
Neck – short
Hands – short metacarpals and phalanges
– clinodactyly
– simian crease
– dermatoglyphics
Feet – gap between first and second toes
Pelvis – hypoplasia – outward lateral flare
Heart – anomolous in 40 per cent
Skin – dry
Hair – sparse
Genitalia – small penis – low fertility

Physical appearance

The physical features of Down's syndrome are known to most people, allowing identification of the vast majority in the newborn period. Obvious floppiness (hypotonia) is a striking and consistent feature in all but a few (see photograph overleaf).

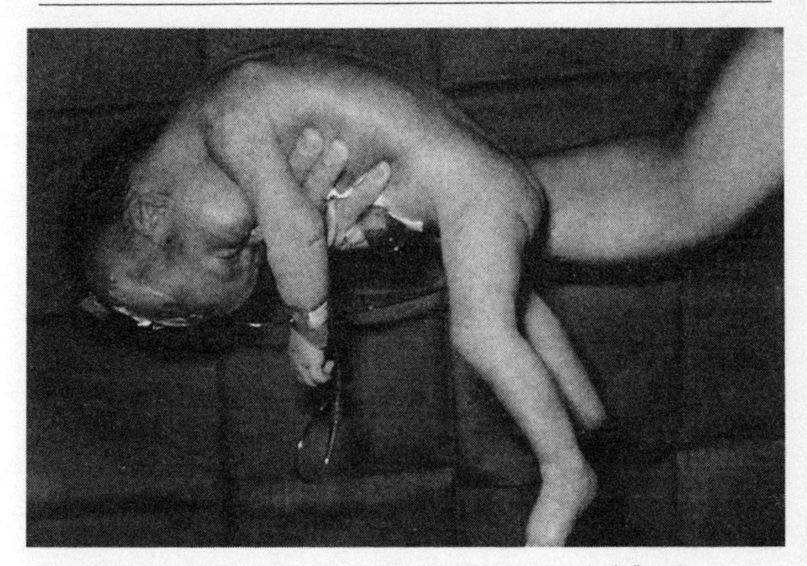

Newborn infant with Down's syndrome, showing marked floppiness (hypotonia).

It should be remembered that there is a wide range of characteristics; few children exhibit them all, and some exhibit only a few. It must be said that in some children the diagnosis can be difficult, and only chromosomal analysis in these cases will exclude or confirm the condition. Modern laboratory techniques allow an answer within 72 hours, although in practice, due to laboratory workload, it often takes longer.

The most consistent features in Down's syndrome are the facial appearance, the skeletal structure leading to short stature, and the developmental anomalies of the heart. The importance of the more common characteristics will be re-addressed in the chapter on health issues.

Mental abilities and structure of the brain

Developmental variations are seen in the brain in Down's syndrome. At the macroscopic level (features seen with the naked eye) such variations can be seen in the pathways that are of importance in processing visual information and memory. These include the anterior commisure, which is

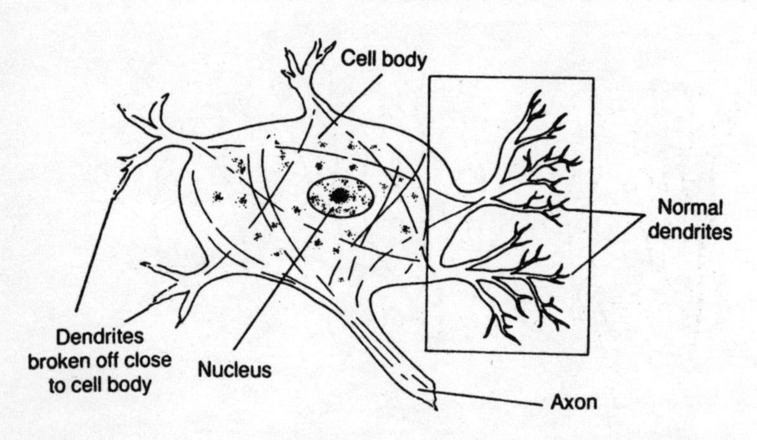

Diagram to show motor nerve cell with the axon (nerve cell body) and dendrites (nerve cell connectors) broken off near to the body of the cell.

smaller in Down's syndrome due to underdevelopment. The commisure represents bands of nerve cells that connect different parts of the brain, and particularly the two limbic systems which are involved in memory function.

The brain is a living information processor made up of millions of nerve cells, each nerve cell communicating with its neighbour through small outgrowths called dendrites. The quality and quantity of these dendrites determines the level of computing and learning ability. At the microscopic level abnormal dendritic processes can be seen in Down's syndrome.

These structural variations, and the malfunction that accompanies them, have a general deleterious effect on higher cerebral function. However, impairment of learning ability has been overemphasised in the past, and the full potential for people with Down's syndrome has only been realised since they have had ready access to education and not been committed to an institutional existence. Overall, there is a very broad range of ability within Down's syndrome, from profound learning difficulties to low/average intelligence. Most children with Down's syndrome have moderate learning difficulties.

Emotional, psychological and social stereotypes have been described, but in practice these descriptions do not bear close

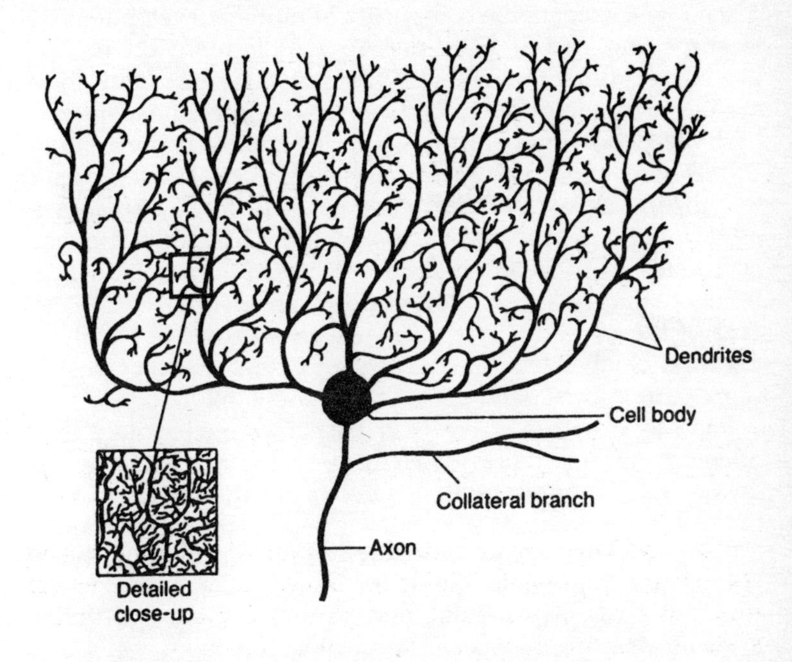

A close-up of a neurone in the cerebellum (one of the motor control cells in the brain), showing the rich network of dendrites normally present and great scope for computing ability!

scrutiny. In general people with Down's syndrome have as many behavioural characteristics as the population as a whole. Comments like 'They love music, don't they?' or 'They are very loving, aren't they?' should not be accepted at face value. These issues will be re-addressed in the chapter on growing up and adult life.

Mechanism of impairment

Dysembryogenesis (when early foetal development goes wrong)

It is one thing to say extra chromosomal material causes Down's syndrome but another thing entirely to understand exactly what the mechanism is. It is clear that dysembryogenesis is an important factor affecting many vital organs. But when one considers the complexity of human development, it is surprising that it does not go wrong more often. The process of differentiation of different cell lines and their organisation into different body organs is ordered or buffered by biofeedback mechanisms which are poorly understood.

In Down's syndrome the extra genetic material seems to lead to a disturbance of the controlling mechanisms, which allows developing organs to become disordered. This mechanism has been referred to as amplified developmental instability. This influence can best be understood by considering that 80 per cent of the manifestations of Down's syndrome are actually minor anomalies seen frequently in isolation in other people (for example Brushfield spots or epicanthic folds).

Recently scientists have paid particular interest to REST, which stands for repressor element-1 silencing transcription factor. REST interacts with a number of other genes to help them regulate normal nerve cell growth and development. This means that REST plays an important part in brain development, neuronal plasticity (that is, versatility in the way the brain can organise itself) and synapse formation (synapses are the 'connector boxes' that join one nerve cell to the next in the circuits through which brain messages are passed). A recent study has suggested that there is a link between malfunction or dysregulation of the REST transcription factor and some of the neurological problems seen in Down's syndrome. Underactivity of REST has been shown to trigger early programmed cell death (known as apoptosis), which could account for the under-development of nerve cells in Down's syndrome, and in particular under-development of the branching and connections of nerve cells.

Cell dysfunction and metabolic disorder

Normal cell function is highly dependent on the activity of enzymes, an enzyme being a biochemical that helps along an essential body process without itself being altered in structure.

One of the first genes to be mapped to the long arm of chromosome 21 was that coding for the enzyme superoxide dismutase (SOD-1). This enzyme is important in the generation of a disruptive process known as lipoperoxidation.

Because of the central importance of lipoperoxidation in the premature ageing process seen in Down's syndrome, and other consequences of cell membrane malfunction (such as faulty neurotransmitter production), it will be dealt with below in some detail.

Other enzyme systems coded on 21q are:

- The production of a protein involved with cataract formation (alpha-A crystal protein) at segment 21q22.
- At 21q21 is an enzyme involved in one stage of glucose production and metabolism (phosfructokinase). Its overactivity may account for a reported excess prevalence of diabetes in people with Down's syndrome.
- An enzyme (cystathionine synthase) that lowers the risk of arteriosclerosis (furred-up arteries), tying in with the fact that people with Down's syndrome have a lower than usual risk of this sort of heart disease.
- Overactive enzyme systems that affect cell membranes appear to be responsible for a number of characteristics, including premature ageing. Alzheimer's disease is very common in Down's syndrome. Those genes coding for familial Alzheimer's disease have been shown to lie adjacent to the protein precursors of an important protein in this disease called amyloid (see Chapter 6 on medical aspects).
- Cell membranes in the body's defence system may also malfunction, making infection and malignancy more common. The augmented risk of leukaemia is associated with a number of genes detailed at www.cancerindex.org. Other oncogenes (cancer susceptibility genes) are in the critical region, including ets-2 at segment 21q22 and an oestrogen-inducible breast cancer gene at 21q 22.3 (BCEI). The significance of this for women with Down's syndrome is not yet clear, as there is no reported excess of that disorder.
- Interferon, a protein with strong anti-viral properties, is also coded for on chromosome 21. Although overproduced because of the gene dosage effect (that is, three rather than two genes are present), it seems far less effective.
- The balance of some neurotransmitters – the biochemicals that are responsible for transporting messages around the

brain and nervous system – is also affected. The precise effect of this is as yet only poorly understood.

Cell malfunction, lipoperoxidation and premature ageing

The body is made up of tiny structures known as cells. Cells are busy and exciting places. They are surrounded by a wall, or cell membrane. They are filled up with a fluid known as cytoplasm, and in the cytoplasm there are a number of structures with a variety of functions. There are energy production plants, production lines and storage areas. The function of each of these structures is determined by genes lying in the control centre in the middle of the cell. The control centre is known as the nucleus and it looks dark under the microscope because that is where the long lines of genes are concentrated on the human chromosomes.

The proteins produced on chromosomal DNA pass out into the cytoplasm, the fluid that fills cells. Here they join with fat (lipid) molecules such as cholesterol and polyunsaturated fatty acids to form the complex lipoprotein structures that make up cell walls, and the smaller power-houses and production lines within the cell that contribute to cell function. Lipoperoxidation disrupts the structure of these lipoproteins and allows oxygen-containing chemicals known as free radicals to become attached to them.

The enzyme called superoxide dismutase (SOD-1, see page 22) has been shown to be 50 per cent more active in people with Down's syndrome. It is responsible for the metabolism of oxygen-free biochemicals and, in so doing, produces oxygen-containing free radicals. It is important that not too many of these free radicals are around in the cell, as many vital cellular processes depend on controlled free-radical metabolism. This is particularly true of the energy production that goes on in tiny intra-cellular power-houses called mitochondria; and of the lipid, protein and glucose release that takes place from another structure known as the endoplasmic reticulum.

Excessive free radical production is at least partly controlled by an enzyme called glutathione peroxidase, along with other catalases (which break down rather than build up) and radical scavengers such as alpha-tocopherol (which collect up and neutralise these free radicals). When these processes are inefficient, the polyunsaturated fatty acids and cholesterol that make up the lipid membrane on the surface of nerve cells become vulnerable.

An increase in lipoperoxidation could explain some of the premature ageing effects seen in Down's syndrome. Pathological studies have shown that, whereas the acquisition of cortical neurones in Down's syndrome is unaffected, the dendritic spines on individual neurones are reduced from the early post-neonatal period onwards. This is due to a premature arrest of growth, so that by the time adult life is reached the dendritic spine deficiency is quite severe. It is through the growth of these dendritic spines that one neurone can communicate with another, thus building up more complex nerve cell circuits, which allow thought, deduction and learning at a higher level.

Studies have shown that abnormal membrane properties are seen in the peripheral tissues of older people with Down's syndrome, and an abnormality of metabolism seen in normal cellular ageing has also been defined. Alzheimer's disease and the high prevalence of cataract are further examples of the analogy that can be drawn between pathological changes in older people with Down's syndrome and what occurs in other humans at a later age.

Any damaging effect of increased SOD-1 activity may be present from early on in foetal life. In the foetal brain it has been shown that SOD-1 activity is increased, with no corresponding increase in the protective effect of glutathione peroxidase activity or alpha-tocopherol, already mentioned as a free radical scavenger and a major lipid anti-oxidant. Therefore brain cells may be more susceptible at an early age, when compensatory mechanisms do not exist. The polyunsaturated fatty acid profile of cell surface membranes has also been shown to resemble those in the brains of older individuals, though the profiles show that the pattern is distorted rather than identical to that of more advanced years.

The metabolism of some vitamins and trace elements

Many parents ask about the value of dietary supplements. While considering aspects of metabolism, it is timely to consider vitamins and trace elements (coenzymes), without which enzymes cannot function efficiently. The following two sections will put their importance into perspective.

Folate metabolism

Although the average serum folate and vitamin B12 levels in Down's syndrome appear to be normal, red cell folate levels have been shown to be very low. There is a corresponding increase in the presence of large red blood corpuscles (macrocytosis) and ultimately a lower serum folate level seen with age. Leukaemia-like nuclear ultrastructural abnormalities in the white blood corpuscles (leucocytes) of people with Down's syndrome have also been shown to be ten times more common than usually found. These nuclear membrane abnormalities do not correlate with serum folate, but both factors are associated with chromosome breakage, which may be partly responsible for the increased risk of malignant change and particularly leukaemia seen in Down's syndrome.

It may thus be of value to monitor red cell folate levels at infrequent intervals, particularly in adult life. If they are shown to be low, folate supplements may be of benefit.

Trace elements

A number of groups have studied trace elements in people with Down's syndrome. One clear message from all these studies is that hair analysis is completely unreliable as a reflection of body metabolism. Many laboratories offer this on a private basis to professionals and parents alike, and they should be avoided.

Glutathione peroxidase is the enzyme, already discussed, that protects against lipo-peroxidation, and it has been shown to need selenium to work efficiently. Early studies had suggested that people with Down's syndrome were plasma selenium deficient. It had been postulated that this leads to a compromise of this protective effect, with a resulting increase in susceptibility to Alzheimer's disease and infection. More recent work has, however, failed to replicate these results, and one Swedish study has shown that plasma selenium is the same as in other people, with red cell selenium actually being higher and reaching adult levels earlier.

Vitamin E has been shown to reduce lipoperoxidation and to have a protective effect when free radicals begin to accumulate in a variety of clinical conditions. However, this research has only been related to short term benefit. Vitamin E has not been shown to offer long term benefit in Down's syndrome. On theoretical grounds it can be argued that there would be some benefit from long term administration of Vitamin E. However, the scientific study that would be needed to demonstrate this would be very difficult to construct. This issue is likely to become clearer over the next few years as the complex biochemistry involved is better understood.

Trace elements have also been studied in red cells, white cells and platelets in people with Down's syndrome. Copper levels have been shown to be consistently raised in all three blood cell types, and it is notable that SOD-1 is copper dependent. Calcium has also been shown to be raised in red cells. Reductions have been seen in the concentrations of zinc and manganese in red cells, of manganese in platelets, with slight reductions of manganese and iron in red and white cells. Titanium has been found in increased levels in most people with Down's syndrome; in the population at large it is not usually raised except in patients with acute myeloid leukaemia. Again, there may be a relationship here between this observation and increased susceptibility to certain types of malignancy.

Other than this, no conclusions can be drawn from these experimental findings; rather than showing a deficiency, low levels might actually represent a beneficial protective compensatory mechanism. Clearly further study is required.

Summary and conclusions

Down's syndrome results from extra chromosomal material present in 50 to 100 genes on the long arm of chromosome 21.

In 95 per cent the cause is trisomy 21, and in about 5 per cent an unbalanced translocation or mosaicism. In 80 per cent of those with trisomy 21 the origin of the extra chromosome is at the time of the first maternal meiosis; that is, in the mother's own foetal life. Genetic factors have been shown to be of importance in relation to vulnerability to non-disjunction at this stage. In the remaining 20 per cent or so the origin is at the stage of maternal meiosis II or paternal meiosis I or II. Environmental agents such as radiation and the contraceptive pill are putative risk factors. Further study is required.

Most of the manifestations of Down's syndrome are minor anomalies seen frequently in isolation in many people. The effect of the increased gene dosage seems to decrease the buffering of potential disorder in developmental pathways. The resulting amplified developmental instability leads to a far greater incidence of these minor anomalies. In the brain and the heart this has an important effect on developmental abilities and general health. Furthermore, disordered enzyme activity leads to an enhancement of biochemical processes, and in particular of lipid peroxidation, which mimic many aspects of premature ageing. In particular, deleterious effects are seen in relation to neurotransmitter formation and the immune process.

3

Incidence, risk of recurrence and antenatal diagnosis

As discussed earlier, the overall incidence of Down's syndrome is 1:660 new borns. The incidence in women under 20 years of age is less than 1:2,000, rising to something like 1:20 at the age of 45. The steepest increment in incidence according to maternal age occurs after the age of 35.

Risk of recurrence

Parents who have had one child with Down's syndrome may wish to know whether it is possible to have another such child.

Overall figures for recurrence are set at about 1 per cent for standard trisomy 21 in women under 35, while after the age of 35 recurrence closely parallels that in the age-related population. When either parent carries a balanced translocation on either the D group or chromosome 22 the chances of recurrence may be as high as 1:5 where the mother is a carrier, or 1:20 where the father is a carrier. For the very rare 21/21 translocation, all subsequent children will have the condition where either parent is a carrier.

After the birth of any child with Down's syndrome, it is therefore advisable for parents to have genetic counselling, which would usually include the drawing up of a very accurate family tree, examination of the parents and a blood test for chromosomal analysis.

Risk of recurrence of Down's syndrome		
Present baby has		*Risk of recurrence*
Standard trisomy 21		
Parents under 30–35		*1 in 100*
Parents over 35		*Depends on age (see page 29)*
Mosaic trisomy 21 and Translocation trisomy 21 where a parent is not a carrier	*Not related to age but so rare that accurate figures are not available*	
Translocation trisomy 21		
D/G translocation (13, 14 or 15/21)		*Between*
When mother is carrier		*1 in 5 and 1 in 10*
When father is carrier		*1 in 20 and 1 in 50*
G/G translocation 21/22		
When mother is carrier		*1 in 5 and 1 in 10*
When father is carrier		*1 in 20 and 1 in 50*
G/G translocation 21/22		
When mother is carrier		*1 in 1*
When father is carrier		*1 in 1*

After Cunningham, C.C., 1988.

Antenatal diagnosis

Amniocentesis

Currently, amniocentesis is offered to most women in Britain aged 35 or over at about 16 weeks' gestation. In amniocentesis a sample of amniotic fluid is obtained and analysed, as it contains foetal cells that can be grown and examined for chromosome abnormality.

The amniocentesis is performed by numbing a small area of skin on the lower abdomen with local anaesthetic, and drawing up the amniotic fluid with a needle and syringe, rather like sampling blood. The risk of miscarriage following amniocentesis is about 1 per cent.

If all women in Britain over 35 had the test, then 7.5 per cent of pregnancies would require amniocentesis and 35 per cent of cases of Down's syndrome would be detected.

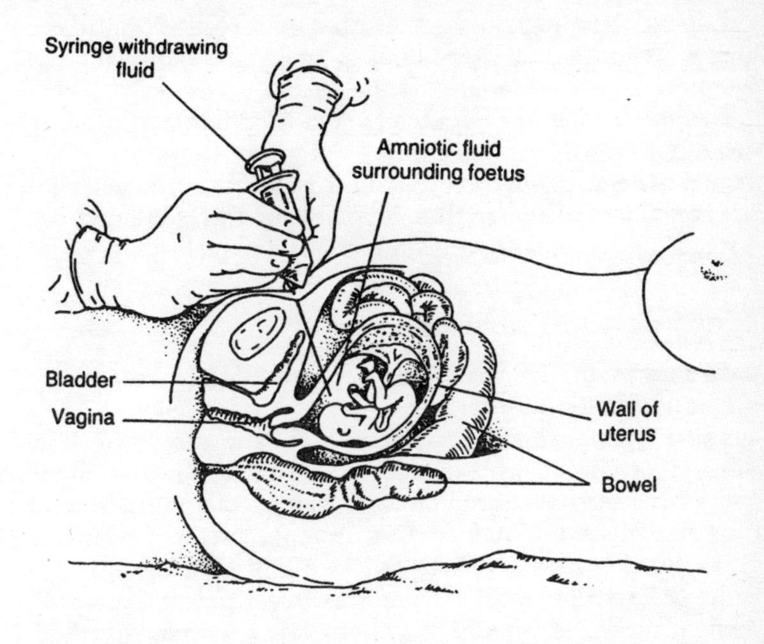

Diagram of how amniocentesis is performed. A needle is advanced through the lower abdominal wall into the uterus. Fluid and cells are withdrawn from the amniotic sac.

Other biochemical tests

It is also known that Down's syndrome in the foetus is associated with low maternal concentrations of alphafoetoprotein, unconjugated oestriol and a high concentration of human gonadotrophin. A risk factor can be derived from these biochemical tests by relating them to maternal age. This offers a new method of screening, known as the 'triple test', which would allow 60 per cent of affected pregnancies to be detected and the overall amniocentesis rate to be reduced to about 5 per cent. This would potentially reduce the number of children born with Down's syndrome in the United Kingdom from about 900 to 350 a year, if those involved wished to terminate the pregnancy. A further biochemical substance known as neutrophil alkaline phosphatase also allows affected pregnancies to be identified with greater accuracy.

Health commissioners in the United Kingdom are currently deciding which method of screening to introduce, their thoughts being centred on cost efficiency and effectiveness. It is essential that all families involved in this screening are offered good counselling on the choices available.

Chorionic villus sampling

A first trimester chorionic villus biopsy offers an alternative method of antenatal diagnosis.

The placenta attaches to the wall of the uterus by little 'fingers' or villi. A probe is inserted via the cervix and one of the villi removed and analysed, giving the same sort of information as is obtained from amniocentesis. Given that currently the quoted risk to the foetus of this test is in the order of 2 to 3 per cent, compared with a 1 per cent risk with amniocentesis, it should probably be reserved for those women with a particularly high risk of recurrence in subsequent pregnancies.

Appropriate counselling should be given before and after both these procedures, and sensitivity will be needed to help with parents' feelings if a positive diagnosis is made, particularly if termination is chosen.

Ultrasound scanning

As the technique of ultrasound scanning has become more sophisticated, so its use has been directed at detecting the presence of Down's syndrome in the developing foetus. For example, if the foetus' head can be examined by ultrasound it is possible to identify the characteristic shape. Another technique is to look for a thickened skinfold at the back of the neck, and a femur (thigh bone) that is shorter than would be expected. If these observations are combined with ultrasound detection of heart abnormalities (which are common in Down's syndrome), the technique is about 80 per cent accurate. As it is very time-consuming, the procedure is not widely available; also, it cannot be performed until the foetus

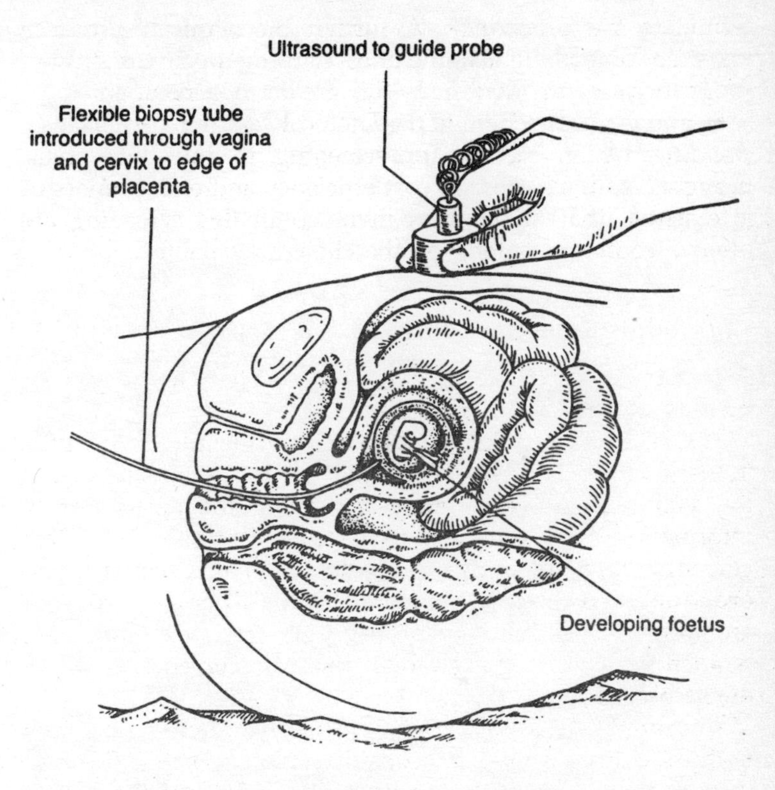

Diagram of how chorionic villus biopsy is performed. A flexible tube is introduced into the vagina through the neck of the womb into the developing chorion. A biopsy is taken.

has developed sufficiently, some time after the 12–14 week stage.

The conclusion is that the use of ultrasound alongside the tissue analysis techniques of amniocentesis and chorionic villus sampling and the biochemical tests such as alphafoeto-protein analysis will allow antenatal diagnosis of Down's syndrome in an ever-growing number of pregnancies, and allow parents concerned an ever greater informed choice. It must be remembered that these clinical methods will only be of real value to parents when they are accompanied by appropriate counselling. There will always be parents who decide not to involve themselves in any method of antenatal diagnosis as they know they would enjoy and value any baby whether it had Down's syndrome or not.

4

Hearing the news

To the happy parents of a newborn baby it comes as an enormous surprise or shock to receive the news that their child may have Down's syndrome. Unless an antenatal diagnosis was made they will have had no warning. The surprise can be even greater if the parents are young, because it is still assumed by the lay-public that babies with Down's syndrome are only born to mothers in their late 30s or older. Although the chance is higher for older mothers, half the women who give birth to a baby with Down's syndrome are younger than 35, with many in their 20s and a small number in their teens.

Despite the very positive changes in attitudes and knowledge about Down's syndrome, it is regrettable that one of the most painful and traumatic experiences many parents of babies with Down's syndrome remember is the manner in which they were told the news by health care professionals, and the kind of support and follow-up they received.

When asked about this experience many parents wanted the following:

- To be told as soon as possible.
- To be told together.
- To be told sympathetically, in private and with respect for their feelings.
- To have the baby present.
- To be given accurate information.
- To be helped to pass on the news to family and friends.

Tell us as soon as possible

What is invariably meant by this is 'Tell us as soon as everybody else is pretty sure'. If there is any doubt over the diagnosis of Down's syndrome it is important that this possibility is discussed with parents at an early stage.

It is to be expected that parents would wish to be included in such discussions as soon as possible. They may have already sensed that something is not quite right soon after delivery; even if they have not actually recognised the signs in the baby's features, the sense that all is not well can be picked up from the attitude of the maternity staff.

The delivery of simple facts as soon as possible will allow parents to dispense with some of the bad and frightening images they may have held previously. This will help them begin to value their baby and realise that they will be able to look after a child with learning difficulties.

Tell us together

The majority of parents want to be told with their partner or a close relative present. A relative or friend can often help parents to recall information and reduce their sense of isolation. Sadly, however, it is still the case that most parents can expect to receive the information without this support.

Value the baby

A significant feature of surveys is that parents want their baby to be present with them when they are told of the diagnosis.

Often the baby is not present at this time. This may appear to parents as if the child is not valued, perhaps because of its condition. It is inevitable that parents are sensitive to the attitudes and behaviour of the maternity and medical staff.

Staff need training on how to handle this counselling and to develop their own positive attitude to disability. However, lack of this knowledge should not prevent staff from being friendly, sympathetic and supportive.

Parents should be encouraged to spend as much time as possible with their new baby, and particularly if the baby is on the special care baby unit. When the baby is present staff should react to it as with any other baby, by holding, rocking and talking.

'The baby was in the room but the doctor never looked at it once.'

'The doctor used to come every day, but she never touched the baby.'

These are two kinds of experience that left parents feeling hurt.

How parents are told is also important. The doctor may not be able to say 'You are very lucky. You have a baby with Down's syndrome', but 'I am terribly sorry, I have some very bad news for you' is too negative. 'I have some news for you which you were not expecting' would be better.

Doctors can also mislead by being too positive. If they propose all kinds of therapy in the wrong light, then parents may think that therapy can 'put the problem right', whereas the real value in the advice therapists give is in encouraging children to reach their full potential (see Chapter 10 for more discussion of this important issue). Doctors should be aware of the values and interpretations that parents attach to such statements, and try to be more factual, balanced and supportive.

Give accurate information and continuing support

In the past parents have often been given the news that their child has Down's syndrome in a way that has left them with some anger, confusion or despair. A number of studies over the years have identified the way in which families would prefer to receive the news. In recent years SCOPE, supported by the Down's Syndrome Association, has established a multidisciplinary working party so that members of the different professions involved might be encouraged to decide on a good standard of practice. This is seen as an important standard, and Primary Care Trusts (formerly health commissioners), are being encouraged to incorporate this standard in their contracts with providers delivering the service. The Community Care Act now specifically states that doctors must introduce families to organisations in the voluntary sector likely to give them support and advice. The campaign steered by SCOPE is known as 'Right from the Start'. Its essential ingredients are as follows:

Parents want accurate information. Even when it is available, they may not be able to absorb it while the situation is still new to them, particularly if the doctor only allows one chance to answer questions.

'I didn't have enough time to take it in.'

'I'd have liked to have seen someone else.'

'I needed to talk to somebody afterwards.'

These are all typical comments from parents.

Giving parents enough time and the chance to talk to someone is a long process, and needs to be planned. Ideally, the first interview should be short, as parents can be upset and may not be able to take much in. The doctor giving the news should be experienced and known to them. It is valuable to have another health care professional, such as a health visitor or social worker, present; they will help re-explain what the doctor has said, to enable the parents to gather their thoughts and questions in time for the next interview with the doctor.

This second interview should take place within 24 hours. At this time parents can be introduced to other sources of information, such as parent support groups like the Down's Syndrome Association. Wherever possible simple written information should be provided to complement what has been said by the doctor.

Some parents may need help on how to pass on the information to other family members and friends. Grandparents can be supportive, although initially they may react by saying that the doctors are wrong and that everything will be all right. Siblings may find it hard to tell friends and teachers; family friends may feel helpless and awkward. Parents have found that a simple and honest approach works best. Health visitors can help by talking to family and friends, but most parents prefer to do it themselves. Some typical experiences are:

> When telling relatives and friends that our much-wanted first child had Down's syndrome we knew that they would find the news sad, and so we broke it gently. Subsequently our son has been accepted and visited by all.

> I am a great believer in being direct with people and not beating about the bush. I was determined to tell everybody – neighbours, friends and casual acquaintances.

> When my little sister was born Mummy and Daddy told me she would need help to learn things, more help than I did. Now she can do lots of things and I take her out to play. I think she is lovely.

Where this general advice and counselling have been followed, surveys show that parents are very satisfied. If parents do not get sensitive help at this critical time, they may fail to seek help later and have difficulty adjusting to their child's disability (see Chapter 9 on growing up). 'By the time the diagnosis was made Stephen was already a part of the family and we could not consider anything other than keeping him with us.'

> I still feel moments of sadness when I think how much help Timmy needs compared to my other grandchildren, but bit by bit I can see some of the tricks in him that the other children have got up to in the past, and I know I am really glad to have him as part of our family.

Even when initial feelings of disappointment and grief are intense, natural improvement comes with time. As parents get to know their new baby better and as they learn more about the prospects of people with Down's syndrome, they grow more confident and begin to enjoy the new arrival's growth and development much as they would any other child. The child with Down's syndrome becomes part of the family and after a few weeks the family begins to laugh again. The next chapter covers some of the key areas that may cause uncertainty and doubt in some parents. Additionally, there are comments and advice from parents who have brought up a child with Down's syndrome.

5

Help with the baby

Feeding

The decision to breastfeed any baby is a very personal one. There is no reason why babies with Down's syndrome should not be successfully breastfed for as long as is necessary; indeed it may help the mother feel close to her baby in the beginning.

> I breastfed Katie for nine weeks. I am sure that breastfeeding creates a wonderful bond between mother and baby, and this is particularly helpful in the case of a handicapped baby.

This is not to deny that there can be problems with breastfeeding a baby with Down's syndrome. The poor muscle tone of the baby can result in the head not being positioned well in relation to the breast, or the lips may make an inefficient seal around the nipple. Furthermore, if the muscle coordination is not as good as it ought to be, the action of swallowing can sometimes be faulty. Certainly, babies with Down's syndrome often seem to have had enough after only a short time – obviously less than they need – and although they often wake and cry for feeds they may just as easily slip back off to sleep without having taken enough.

When beginning to feed it is therefore important for the baby to be held fairly upright, and in particular to have the head supported. It should be checked that the tongue is not sticking to the roof of the mouth; for a baby to suckle successfully and get adequate milk, the nipple (or teat, if bottle feeding) must be on the tongue, not under it. Swallowing can be assisted by supporting the baby's lower jaw with the fingers and moving it in a rhythmical manner; this also has the advantage of improving the lip seal.

It is best not to hurry the feed. Babies with Down's syndrome often feed very slowly indeed. As Harriet's mum said, 'Harriet suckled weakly at first, so I kept her alert and awake by tickling her cheeks, chin and feet.'

The baby may also fall asleep at intervals during the feed. It is worthwhile unwrapping the baby, withdrawing the breast or bottle, and changing the nappy before and during the feed.

> I managed to breastfeed for four days, but Timothy was a very lazy feeder and it was becoming obvious that he might lose weight. I decided that I would be much happier bottle feeding him as then I could see how much he was getting. Although this was rather difficult, Timothy began to gain weight.

Temperature control

In babies with Down's syndrome in particular, the body's heat-regulating mechanism does not always work during the early weeks of life, which may in turn contribute to an increased susceptibility to colds and bronchial infections. It is therefore important to ensure that the baby is warm enough, but not too warm.

The bedroom should not feel too cold at night-time, and it should be draught-free. An all-in-one sleeping suit or sleeping bag is useful, as cot blankets and covers can often get kicked off. It is worth remembering that two thin layers of clothing are better than one thick one, and one of the layers can be removed if the baby gets too hot. In cold weather a hat should be worn, even indoors if the house is cold; the head is one of the greatest sources of heat loss.

Skin care

The skin of a baby with Down's syndrome can tend to be very dry. Massaging the skin all over with a little baby oil will help, and will have the advantage of stimulating the baby as well. Baby oil can also be put in the bathwater.

Alternatively, a little moisturising cream, e.g. Creme E45, or unperfumed cold cream can be rubbed into the skin every day. This will prevent drying and cracking. Allergic reactions to the creams are rare.

Tongue control

Because of the poor muscle coordination, the baby may need special attention to help control the tongue. Playing games such as pulling faces and making noises will all help the child exercise the face and tongue muscles, and will also help with early sounds and, later, with speech. For example, a game could be made of pushing in the tongue over and over again.

As a blocked nose encourages an open mouth and a protruding tongue, an effort should be made to keep it clear.

Developing movement

From the very first weeks after birth the baby should receive lots of encouragement to move. This can be achieved by all sorts of means. For example:

- By bringing the baby into contact with a wide variety of contrasting surfaces – hard and soft, rough/prickly and smooth.
- By handling the baby a lot – with lots of cuddles, tickles, hugs and massage.
- By playing with the fingers and toes.

A fuller list of more detailed activities is given on pages 43–4 of this chapter.

Hand/eye coordination

As with any other baby, hand/eye coordination can be developed by providing the baby with Down's syndrome with things to see, touch, feel and listen to, whether in the pram, baby-chair, cot or on the floor. For example, brightly coloured mobiles and musical toys provide good visual interest.

> Before our son was born I heard a programme on the radio in which a mother described the achievements of her little

girl with Down's syndrome. Our determination to teach our son everything that an ordinary child does naturally has given us endless rewards – the whole family has gained from helping our slow learner.

Damola, our grandson, is the light of our lives. It was a shock to us all when he was born and we were told he had Down's syndrome, but he is now a bright adventurous child going through the 'terrible twos' stage. We are proud of how our daughter and her husband have managed.

Activities

The stimulation of babies from an early stage is an enjoyable introduction to the process of learning. Some suggestions are as follows:

- Blowing on all parts of the baby's body. Tickling, rubbing, patting and gently prodding the baby. Rolling the baby around.
- Lying the baby down naked on a coarse woollen blanket or on crackly paper so that the nerves of the body receive the feel of something different. This can be particularly valuable as an incentive to movement, especially as the sound of the noisy paper is a reward in itself.
- Putting the baby close to the bottom of the cot to encourage pushing against it.
- Placing the baby face down and holding some bright noisy object in front of the eyes and above the head. This will encourage lifting the head to exercise the neck muscles.
- Whistling and singing, using odd sounds that suddenly lapse into a peaceful silence. Any sounds that produce stretches or arching of the back, wriggles or happy twisting.
- Positioning little bells in the cot, not only near the baby's hands but also near (or even on) the feet; this will encourage the baby to kick out more frequently and purposefully. If the bells are placed in the side of the cot the baby may even learn to use alternate limbs.
- Carrying the baby in a sling. In this way the baby is rocked, lowered, lifted and turned in the course of mother's

activity. It will also stimulate the sense of balance and reinforce the feeling of being loved and being part of everything.

- Teasing the baby into making turning, stretching and bending movements by holding some desired object a slight distance away. By making an effort to reach it the baby will learn that effort has its rewards.
- If the baby seems to be making no attempt to crawl, putting a large rolled-up towel in the bath may help. This comfortable bulge will support the chest and abdomen while leaving the limbs free to dangle in the supporting water. Splashing in this position is very close to the movements of crawling.
- It is enjoyable to get down to the same level as the baby to play. By pushing the soles of their feet against the baby's, parents can encourage more active leg movement. The baby can be pulled to standing from this position, or the parent's legs can be used as a ramp to climb.
- Making the baby itch with curiosity by doing something secretive nearby, or clattering about unseen, can make the baby want to overcome the physical stumbling block and get up and find out what is going on.

One parent's view

For me the beginnings of bringing up a slow learner (I prefer this label as it is more hope inspiring than the word handicapped) were not easy. Although the books on baby play were helpful, I still had to feel my way through, especially as my daughter was my first child.

I would let her be close to me a lot; for example, I carried her in a sling, or I wheeled her around the house in a small cot. I propped her up in a slanting chair placed near me on top of the sink or table (ideal for the two of us to look, listen, touch and babble).

I would not let her doze too much, and would not accept this tendency on her part simply as part of 'the condition'. I found that if I made something stand out for her, if I selected for her what she might not have been able to select herself from an overwhelming setting, she showed little sign of tiredness and switching off. Her eyes became alert, her body more tense and her little head less likely to sink loosely into the back of her neck. However, I still respected her need for some switching-off time, as indicated by her remote gaze.

Apart from general babycare, I tried to change the routines. For example I changed her in different places; a bath could be taken in the sink, or with Dad, or in the swimming pool; physical play could occur on a puffy eiderdown or a rough mat.

Parents should not feel compelled to spend a set amount of time in play each day; running a household, particularly if there are other children, is a time-consuming business. Research has shown that as long as the relationship between parents and child is a loving one, then the quality of play and interaction will be good. The quality is probably far more important than the quantity.

Safe, bright and interesting modern toys offer great scope for good quality play. They are designed to delight, provoke and provide enjoyment. If cradle toys are fixed where the feet and knees can kick them, or where the elbows push out, movement is encouraged. It is helpful to use cradle toys made of materials other than plastic, and covered with different textures. Different colours can be used, from pinks and blues to glittering golds and silvers. Wooden toys with clippety-clop sounds, or clicks and clanging cymbals, instead of the usual bell and beady sounds, add variety to experience. Children can be surprised by hanging up a fat balloon, tiny beads, a closed plastic water bag for squeezing, a piece of chocolate, or a mirror. An idea of object permanence can grow out of covering things suddenly and then letting them reappear.

In short, as parents we decided to be on her side, and not make behaviour training our first concern. Looking back, this seems like a daring attitude to have taken, but my now ten-year-old daughter shows me that for her this must have been right.

6

Medical aspects of Down's syndrome

When poor health in Down's syndrome arises it is usually due to maldevelopment of particular organs, or as a result of processes akin to premature ageing or disordered immunity. This chapter will look at specific health problems, and will outline what can be done. Particular emphasis will be placed on heart disease, as this is the commonest cause of poor health in young people with Down's syndrome.

General considerations

Although it does not offer a threat to good health, the skin of children with Down's syndrome is often of concern to parents. The skin tends to be drier than in other children, with a particular tendency to seborrhoeic dermatitis (a dry flakiness or crusting) of the scalp. In cold windy weather the face may become very sore and chapped. The best remedy is the prudent use of a barrier cream, and the addition of oilatum emollient to the bathwater.

Dryness of the skin in some areas of the body can be very marked, with the formation of hyperkeratotic areas (areas of thickened horny skin). Up to 75 per cent of individuals with Down's syndrome will show these, the commoner sites being on the back of the upper arm, including the elbow.

About half the people with Down's syndrome have reddened pimply eruptions, particularly on the trunk, upper thigh and buttock. These areas are actually a dense collection of collagen around normal hair follicles, often with some surrounding inflammation. They can become infected, leading to painful boil and abscess formation, though this is avoidable with appropriate washing and hygiene.

Young people with Down's syndrome also have an increased tendency to alopoecia areata and totalis (patchy bald areas which may come and go, and in some very rare cases total baldness). Vitiligo (areas of reduced skin pigmentation) is also seen more frequently than expected. There are known associations between these disorders and circulating autoantibodies (chemicals produced by the immune system that attack tissues in the body rather than combating infection), although the exact mechanism is unknown. As will be seen in the section on thyroid disorders, it is of interest that people with Down's syndrome have an increase in thyroid autoantibody production too.

As in many children with a disorder of the central nervous system (the brain and spinal cord), there is often relatively poor control of skin blood supply. This often leads to mottling of the skin, in a pattern that corresponds with the pattern of blood vessels. This is particularly evident in the neonatal period, and is known as cutis marmorata. At any age this may lead to the extremities, and in particular the feet and hands, appearing very cold. This rarely seems to give the children themselves any particular concern, but it seems appropriate to use thicker socks on these occasions and make a particular effort to keep gloves on (not always an easy task).

Tears are produced by the lachrymal gland, which lies at the inner end of each pair of eyelids. If the tears do not spill over the lower lid on to the cheek, they normally pass down a tunnel, known as the naso-lachrymal duct, to the nose; this is why the nose often needs blowing after crying. Imperfect canalisation of the naso-lachrymal duct is common in Down's syndrome. This leads tears to run down the face rather than into the nose, and may be particularly noticeable in cold and windy weather. The eye may become dry, and infection may lead to a crusting of green-coloured matter around the eyes. Wiping the eyes with saline is the best solution, but if the whites of the eyes become inflamed (conjunctivitis) a course of antibiotic drops may be needed. In the long term, probing of the duct under a short anaesthetic usually relieves the problem.

As in most toddler children, those with Down's syndrome often have a continually runny nose as they pass from one 'cold' (upper respiratory-tract infection) to the next, particularly in winter months. At times the nasal discharge is clear, and at others green or yellow (mucopurulent). Antibiotics should probably be reserved for definite evidence of middle-ear infection (otitis media), lower respiratory tract infection (bronchitis or pneumonia) or when nasal discharge persists for a week. There is generally only a need to take children to the doctor for advice on this when they are clearly ill in themselves, with a persistent high temperature, when they are listless and cannot be bothered to do anything, or if they are tending to pull at one ear. Irritant coughs at night due to catarrh can be eased by the use of sympathomimetic agents which dry up secretions, such as pseudoephedrine.

An irregular dentition is quite common in Down's syndrome, with missing teeth or abnormalities in tooth shape and position. This is another example of poorly canalised developmental pathways (see Chapter 2), leading to an increased variation of normal. Although the incidence of dental caries is lower than in the general population, periodontal (gum) disease is more prevalent. This may be another effect of relatively poor immunity, and makes it particularly important for young children with Down's syndrome to learn about dental hygiene and good teeth cleaning in particular.

The neurology of Down's syndrome – motor abilities

Hypotonia (poor muscle tone) is one of the main features of Down's syndrome. A relative deficiency of excitatory neurotransmitters such as 5-hydroxytryptamine (serotonin), underdevelopment of the cerebellum (one of the motor control centres in the brain), and a generally poor level of dendritic development (see Chapter 2) all play a part. The result is that the resting activity in the neural apparatus in muscles (the muscle spindles and their connections with the spinal cord and brain) is 'set' at too low a level, and muscle tone, particularly in the axis (head and trunk) is poor. Limb tone may be relatively normal, and power at any age is good. The hypotonia generally resolves with age, but there are few adults with Down's syndrome who are not a little hypotonic. This particularly shows itself in the lower leg, and people with Down's syndrome often have flat feet with a tendency for the ankle to bend outwards (known as the valgus position).

Normal motor development in the first year of life establishes the upright posture. This allows children mobility, with their mouth, hands, eyes and ears free to explore the exciting world and build on their learning experience. Primitive reflexes are imprinted on the central nervous system, from the spinal cord through to brain stem level, helping progress through a series of developmental steps. For example, the asymmetrical tonic neck reflex ensures that every time a baby turns its head a hand appears before the eyes as a cupid-like posture is adopted. The baby quickly learns that the hand that keeps appearing in front of the eyes is part of its own body. This learning is reinforced and consolidated by the information received from the eyes, along with tactile information as the baby starts to explore with its mouth.

A number of studies on Down's syndrome have shown that the primitive reflexes in some children persist for longer than expected, while in others they disappear prematurely. Cliff Cunningham's researchers working at the Hester Adrian Research Centre in Manchester showed that intervention before six weeks of age could maintain the presence of the stepping reflex and facilitate early walking. This emphasises that the reciprocal pattern of walking is actually imprinted at a spinal cord level. Interestingly, those children with enhanced cognitive skills (growing intelligence) seemed to fare worst on motor skills. This implies that the two areas of learning are separate.

Conflicting results have been reported in relation to the persistence of primitive reflexes, and the relationship motor development has to general development. This serves to emphasise that there are as many differences between people with Down's syndrome as there are in the population as a whole, and that those differences should receive as much emphasis as the similarities.

Physio- and occupational therapists can be very helpful to families in advising them on what to incorporate in play in order to encourage the next developmental stage. Particular attention should be paid to positioning and seating.

The limitation of motor performance in the older child with Down's syndrome comes from an inherent and sometimes severe dyspraxia. This means that, although the muscles have power and strength to carry out movement, it is often laboured or clumsy.

People are able to move because they know what a movement feels like. When Tim Henman hits a winning volley he does not have to say to himself that he must pull the racket backwards, transfer his weight on to the back foot, fix the shoulder girdle muscles and so on: he does it because his brain has controlled that movement many times before and is quite capable of building up and processing information from the eyes, ears and sensory equipment in his arms and legs about exactly where his body is in space and exactly what he must do to perform the movement he wishes. In the same way, this is just how we, in a rather less spectacular manner, scratch our noses or put a spoonful of food in our mouths; at first by trial and error, and then with an increasing degree of accuracy.

In Down's syndrome there appears to be a significant problem with this integration of sensory information and the coordination of motor output. The child will be quite aware of what is to be achieved, and will have the equipment to achieve it, but be quite unable to get the movement together. The feedback and integration pathways are relatively inefficient. In addition, many with Down's syndrome have slow reaction times, a poor ability to dissociate movement (i.e. make one hand do a different thing from the other, as in playing the piano) and difficulty with anticipatory skills and sequencing where the object of the movement is not static (such as hitting a ball). It is probably reaction time, rather than a lack of feeling, that causes children with Down's syndrome to be slow to remove themselves from pain. In these circumstances hot radiators or fingers in a closing door become potentially hazardous and emphasise the need for others to be careful with their advice and with what they do.

These problems of integrating feedback information, and the constant need for adjustment and correction in motor control, are particularly evident in speech. Motor performance in Down's syndrome cannot be regarded as slow normal, but as different (deviating as it does from the usual developmental pathway). This is important for therapists to remember as they devise an individual's intervention programme. For example, a significant proportion of young people with

Down's syndrome develop a stammer. This is a common finding anyway in the general population, with 1 in 20 boys of school entry age showing a speech dysfluency of this type. In Down's syndrome it can be persistent, but a speech therapist can offer many ways to help this.

Awkward walking or running is often obvious in Down's syndrome. It is common for the most severely disabled to walk with a fairly stiff-legged gait, and many walk in a valgus (tilting outwards) position at the ankle, with everted (pointed outwards) fore-feet. Where this is severe the question of a spinal cord problem due to atlanto-axial dislocation arises (see later in this chapter). However, the presentation of this more serious disorder would be of a deteriorating stiff-legged gait, usually accompanied by bladder or bowel disturbance. In the more severely disabled this may be difficult to define, and where doubt exists an MRI scan of the lower brain stem and upper cervical spine needs to be obtained. For the vast majority the observed posture will be no more than the expression of the underlying brain malfunction, and the gait will improve with the sensible use of heel cups and supportive footwear.

Ear abnormality and audiological assessment

Audiological assessment, hearing tests

Any child who has developmental delay, hypotonia and delayed speech and language requires careful assessment to identify the cause of the speech delay and make sure appropriate services are organised. From time to time children are seen where this has not been carried out 'because the medical diagnosis is obvious'; that is, further assessment is not carried out because it is assumed that the Down's syndrome is the sole cause of the delay. But at least half of children with Down's syndrome will have significant hearing problems.

When sound arrives at the ear, it is funnelled down a canal called the external ear, where it falls on the eardrum (tympanic membrane). The drum vibrates and sends a series of waves of vibration, in time with the sound waves, down a string of three little bones (ossicles) – called the hammer, anvil and stirrup (malleus, incus and stapes). The stirrup is attached

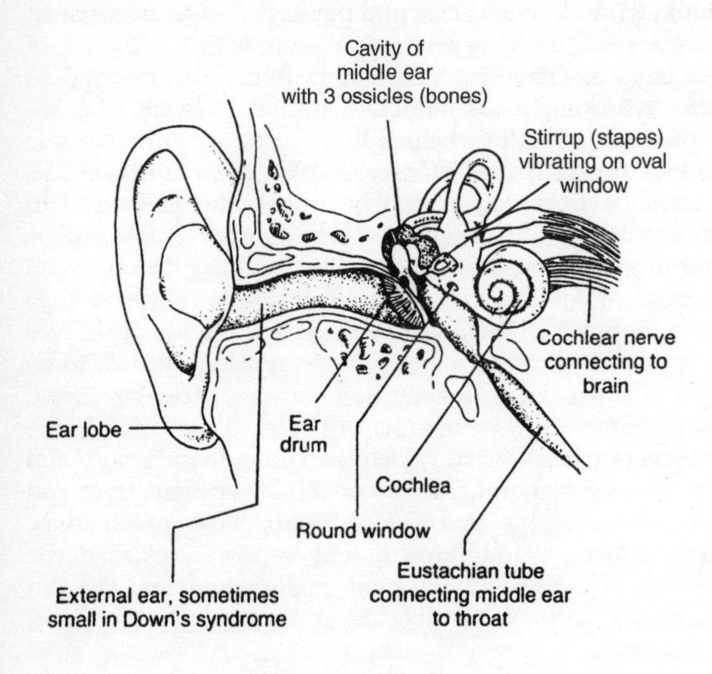

Diagram of external, middle and internal ear.

to a membrane which forms a window, through which lies the inner ear. The cavity containing the ossicles, between the eardrum and the oval window, is known as the middle ear; it is connected to the back of the nose by the Eustachian tube. The middle ear is normally full of air. This is why when ears 'pop' they can be made to feel comfortable again by holding the nose and blowing out hard against a closed throat, forcing air back up the tube into the middle ear. As the stirrup rocks against the oval window, the vibrations are sent into the inner ear, again in time with the sound that originally formed them.

The inner ear contains an organ called the cochlea; it contains specialised hair-cells that waft in a fluid called endolymph. The pattern of vibration formed by the stirrup is picked up by the cochlea hair-cells and transmitted to the brain via the eighth cranial nerve. The temporal lobes of the brain then 'decode' the sound message and make sense of it.

Hearing loss due to a problem in either the external or middle ear is known as conductive deafness; hearing loss due to a problem with the cochlea or its central connections is known as sensorineural or nerve deafness. Conductive loss can often be treated, and can be more often helped with hearing aids; nerve deafness is usually permanent, and is more difficult to help.

The hearing loss in Down's syndrome is sensorineural in 20 per cent of cases, and this incidence increases with age. Up to 50 per cent of people with Down's syndrome will at some stage have a conductive deafness, partly due to susceptibility to developing an accumulation of thick fluid within the middle ear space. This is called otitis media with effusion (OME) or more commonly 'glue ear'. Infection of this glue-like fluid can occur and is often recurrent. (see below). One study showed an excessive accumulation of wax in the external ear to be the commonest otological complication of Down's syndrome (31 per cent, versus 14 per cent in other children). Hearing loss in these children averaged 24 decibels (dB). This shows how important it is to be on the lookout for a readily remediable problem.

All children with Down's syndrome should have a formal audiological assessment in infancy and at regular intervals during childhood, the intervals depending on the initial findings. If remedial treatment is not undertaken, a child with hearing loss may develop the secondary problem of poor auditory perception at a cortical level (that is, the brain failing to make sense of what it hears because it has had so little experience of sound, which may in turn affect speech and learning).

One means of assessing how effective any treatment is is to carry out a controlled trial, the results of one form of treatment being compared to those in another group of children (the controls) who have no, or another form of, treatment. It is essential that the results are assessed in an unbiased way, and for this reason the assessor is often not told what treatment has been given (this is a single-blind controlled trial). Sometimes, if the pharmacist has matched the active treatment with a period on a placebo that is identical in appearance but inactive, neither the family nor doctor know what treatment is given (in this case it is a double-blind controlled trial). It is only when these strict scientific rules are followed that we can be absolutely sure that something is effective. Proper assessment is essential, as many treatments are uncomfortable, have side-effects or carry an expense. This subject will be returned to in Chapter 10, on hopes and fears.

There have been a number of controlled trials of treatment for conductive deafness due to middle ear effusions (a collection of fluid). It is generally agreed that surgical treatment is indicated where there are bilateral effusions, a persistent subjective hearing loss, a bilateral 25-decibel loss over two or more frequencies, or a bilateral flattening of the tympanogram (measuring how easily the ears 'pop'). A number of studies have shown that adenoidectomy associated with myringotomy (making a hole in the drum to let out the fluid) and the insertion of grommets (tiny plastic washers) result in the quickest resolution of both middle ear effusions and infection, and the fastest return of hearing. The majority of the benefit seems to come from the adenoidectomy rather than the insertion of grommets; the long-term effects of grommets are yet to be discerned. One study showed a 40 per cent incidence of a degree of tympanosclerosis (scarring of the drum) after 12 months and a 70 per cent incidence after 21 months. We now know tympanosclerosis has a minimal effect on hearing and is functionally unimportant. The problem with grommets is that in children with Down's syndrome they can be difficult to insert, as the external ear canal is narrow and it is therefore difficult to get the grommet into the correct position. Also as a result of the narrow canal, water tends to remain in the canal after bathing and infect the grommet. Recurrent infections of the grommet are not an uncommon problem in children with Down's syndrome.

There have been no controlled studies to date on the best treatment of hearing loss in children with Down's syndrome. Where the strict selection criteria cited above exist, adenoidectomy is probably still of benefit, but a surgical approach must be complemented by the skilful provision of hearing aids, with appropriate counselling of parents and teachers in their use. A 2002 German study on hearing defect in 102 children with Down's syndrome showed that 56 per cent had a hearing

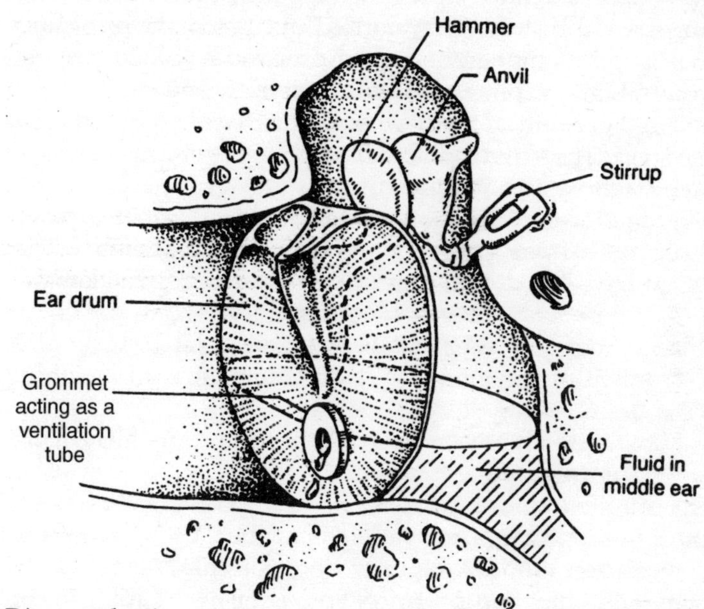

Diagram showing grommets inserted into ear drum draining middle ear.

problem. Of these children, 88 per cent had a conductive hearing loss, 5 per cent had a sensory hearing loss and 7 per cent had a combined conductive and sensorineural loss. The majority (88 per cent) of the conductive loss was of mild or moderate degree.

Snoring, a common problem in Down's syndrome, may also be an indication for adenotonsillectomy. Stradling and colleagues from Oxford published a study on 61 snoring children without Down's syndrome. They found that 61 per cent had important degrees of sleep hypoxia (low blood oxygen) and 65 per cent had abnormally disturbed sleep. Many showed daytime sleepiness, hyperactivity, aggression, learning difficulties, restless sleep and odd sleeping positions. Adenotonsillectomy resolved the hypoxia, sleep disturbance and attendant symptoms for the majority. Marcus and colleagues looked at 53 children with Down's syndrome from California and found a very similar percentage of them (60 per cent) had sleep-related upper airways obstruction as assessed from parental history. They carried out overnight recordings using a polysomnogram (which measures blood oxygen concentration, respiratory rate, heart rate and so on) and found 100 per cent of them carried a degree of abnormality at some stage. They concluded that parental history may serve to under-diagnose (or at times over-diagnose) a problem, and where significant suspicion of sleep-related upper airways obstruction existed, polysomnogram was the definitive test. Interestingly, they found that upper airways obstruction was not the cause of a rise in blood carbon dioxide in all the children. Some of them had problems related to under-development of the lungs, or under-stimulation of breathing via the brain during sleep.

A number of approaches is available for management. Time is a very useful treatment and it is often advisable to wait up to six months before advocating any specific intervention. Topical decongestants and steroids may be a useful temporising measure. While local infection subsides, airways get bigger and breathing control mechanisms during sleep improve.

In Down's syndrome, too, adenotonsillectomy is then probably the treatment of choice. However, careful assessment would be required preoperatively, as the presence of abnormal pharyngeal anatomy in Down's syndrome may predispose to postoperative hypernasality (a tendency to speak through the nose). If the problem persists after this, nasal continuous positive airways pressure (CPAP) has been shown in a number of series to be a very effective treatment for sleep-related upper airways obstruction. This does, however, involve wearing a mask overnight, often difficult to achieve in children with Down's syndrome.

Eye problems and visual assessment

Eye problems are probably even more common than ear abnormalities. The majority of children with Down's syndrome show a degree of hypermetropia (long-sightedness), though this is often not of a degree that needs correction. Up to 20 per cent may show myopia (short-sightedness) and a smaller percentage astigmatism (an irregular lens, leading to focusing problems in different planes). Screening in infancy should be carried out, with appropriate follow-up. When corrective lenses in the form of spectacles or contact lenses are required, appropriate counselling and support should be offered.

Refractive error may be accompanied by strabismus (squint), and corrective surgery is sometimes required. A head tilt may be a clue to the presence of a squint. In up to 5 per cent of cases, congenital cataracts (see Chapter 2) may occur, requiring removal of the diseased lens and the provision of corrective spectacles. Slit lamp examination reveals lens opacities in up to 50 per cent of children with Down's syndrome, this percentage increasing with age. But in the vast majority of cases these are not found in the visual axis and do not interfere with sight.

Specific health problems

Congenital heart and lung disease

Although only one organ, the heart has two distinct halves. The right heart receives blood from the great veins in the body, collects it in the right atrium and then passes it through the tricuspid valve into the right ventricle, a big muscular chamber that pumps blood through the lung (pulmonary) circulation to pick up oxygen. Blood is then returned to the left heart, again to an atrium first and then through the mitral valve into the even larger and more muscular left ventricle, which has the task of pumping the oxygen-laden blood to all the tissues in the body. Normally the right heart and pulmonary circulation is a low pressure system whilst the left heart and the general (systemic) circulation is a high pressure system.

There is normally no connection between the two sides of the heart. If there is an abnormal connection, blood will tend to flow from the high pressure left to the lower pressure right side of the heart. As this blood has already been to the lungs, the child will still normally be pink. This abnormal flow of blood from one side of the heart to the other is known as a shunt. As more blood than usual is now in the lung blood vessels, the pressure in the right side of the heart will go up. It is possible for the pressure to rise so much that it is actually

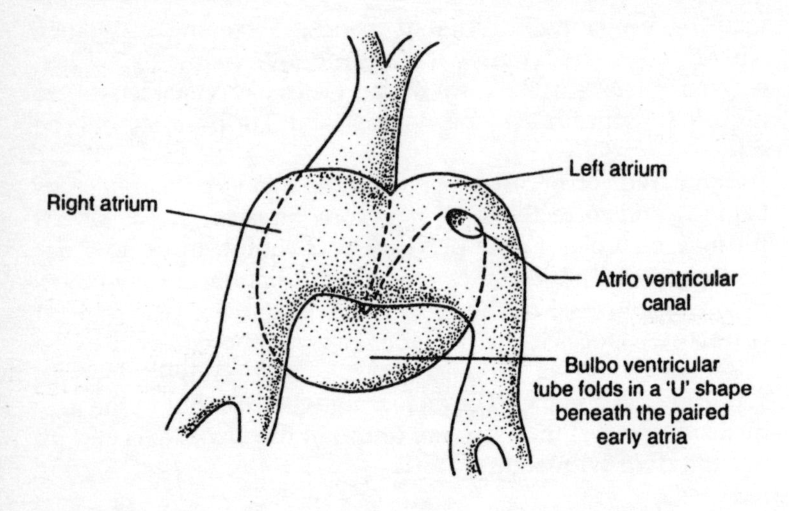

Diagram of heart development at 4 weeks after conception. Paired tubes on each side have fused to form early right and left atria. Tubes in the midline have joined together and begin to fold to form the bulbo ventricular tube.

above that in the left side of the heart; this will cause blood to flow in the opposite direction (reverse shunting) and, because it has yet to visit the lungs, it will be low on oxygen, and the child will appear blue (cyanosed).

In the developing foetus the heart starts out as a tube. The tube folds so that the left heart comes to lie slightly above and in front of the right heart. Outgrowths of tissue known as endocardial cushions grow into the cavity of the primitive heart and form the dividing walls (septa) between the two atria and ventricles, a seat for the two valves, an anchor point for the wall that separates the two atria (interatrial septum) and the wall that separates the two ventricles (interventricular septum).

About 40 per cent of children with Down's syndrome have congenital heart disease, and the commonest form is the atrioventricular canal defect. The endocardial cushions are incompletely formed, leading to deficient septa between the atria and ventricles and inefficient mitral and tricuspid valves. Many defects allow initial left-to-right shunting of blood, with a gradual build-up of pulmonary arterial pressure, facilitated

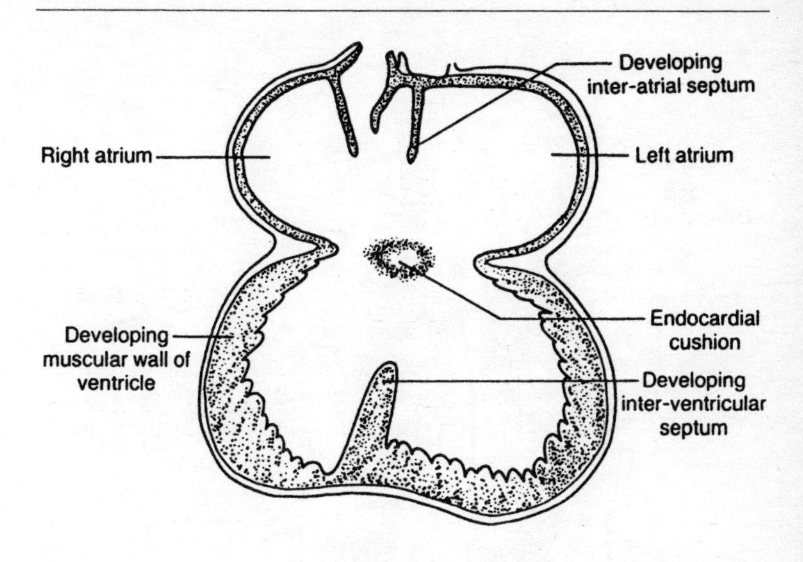

Two weeks later atria and ventricles are formed and the septa grow towards the endocardial cushions which form the seat for the valves.

on occasions by abnormal pulmonary blood vessels (see below). After some time the resulting pulmonary arterial hypertension (high blood pressure) will reverse the shunt and lead to cyanotic heart disease.

Heart disease may present in the form of a murmur picked up at a routine newborn medical examination; by paroxysmal coughing; or by the presence of breathlessness, particularly at feeding times in the early months or with exercise later. Episodes of pallor and sweating in babies often herald the onset of cardiac failure. About 5 per cent of children with Down's syndrome who have congenital heart disease will have no murmurs initially, and their disease will go unnoticed until the onset of cyanosis, by which time it may be too late for corrective surgery.

For this reason routine echocardiography at a regional centre is recommended for all newborn babies with Down's syndrome. This involves checking the heart with a sort of ultra-sound device similar to those used during pregnancy. Where an abnormality is identified, further assessment of the functional consequences will be defined by means of cardiac

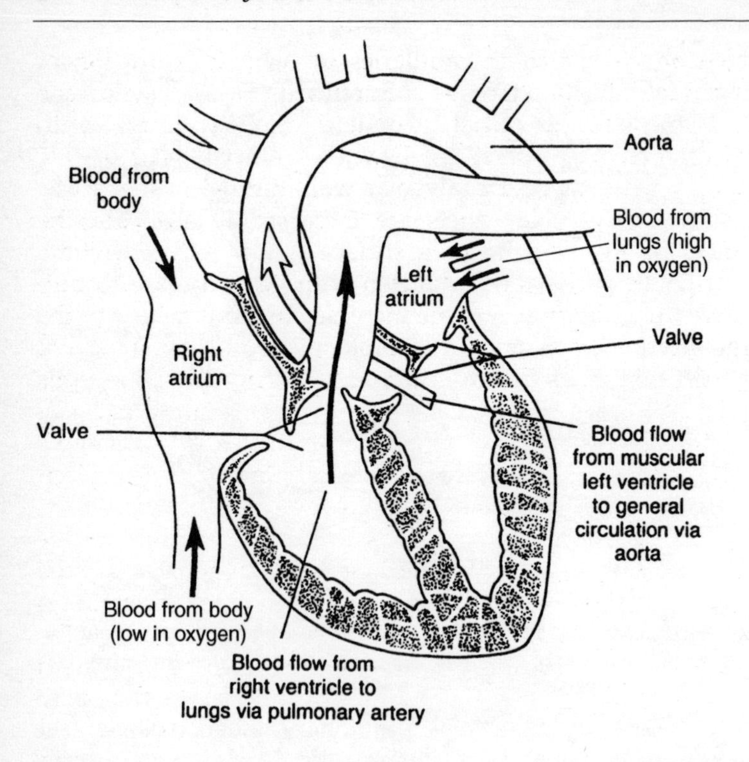

Complete heart development with separate right and left atria and and right and left ventricles.

catheterisation. The information this yields will allow a rational decision on the timing of intervention to be taken. Cardiac catheterisation involves feeding a small tube along a vein or artery to the heart and measuring the pressures in the different chambers. Dye may also be injected so that the anatomy can be defined using X-rays.

Congenital heart disease accounts for 30 to 35 per cent of deaths in Down's syndrome, and the mortality is highest in the first two years of life. Chest infections account for approximately the same number of deaths, but it is conceivable that a congenital cardiac defect may contribute to some of these cases.

The lung consists of millions of tiny air-cells called alveolae, which are very rich in capillaries to help the diffusion of oxygen into the blood. Some children with Down's syndrome are born with hypoplastic (underdeveloped) lungs, with structural changes specific to Down's syndrome. The double capillary network on the alveolar wall, normal in foetal life, persists. The alveolar ducts are increased in size, but the number of alveolae and their surface area is reduced. These abnormalities predispose children with heart disease to pulmonary hypertension, and the increased blood flow due to the large arteriovenous shunt also predisposes to chest infection. An inefficient body defence (immune) system may add to this tendency.

A decision needs to be made, irrespective of the child's ability, on whether to attempt surgical correction. The decision-making process should involve a lot of discussion between the parents and medical team, to share knowledge and weigh up the advantages and disadvantages of the different options available in individual cases. Sometimes temporary solutions can be found such as 'banding' the pulmonary artery. Here the surgeon applies a band around the vessel, making it far more difficult for the blood to flow to the lungs. It then takes the easier route into the left heart and on to the general circulation, while the lungs are protected from the excessive volumes of blood that lead to secondary pulmonary hypertension. The more definitive corrective surgery can then be carried out at a later date.

A conservative policy, using purely medical as opposed to surgical treatment, guarantees a far higher rate of childhood survival. Affected people are likely to live on to their third or fourth decade, when death inevitably occurs due to cardiac failure or concomitant lung disease. Surgical treatment still carries mortality (but this is now less than 5 per cent and is no higher in children with Down's syndrome than in other children). Even after surgery there may be a residual anomaly, yet surgery remains the only chance to avoid the crippling pulmonary vascular disease.

The mainstay of medical treatment remains digoxin and diuretics for cardiac failure, beta-blockers for cyanotic attacks due to pulmonary artery spasm, and antibiotic prophylaxis to cover dental procedures so that bacterial endocarditis (infection of the heart) may be avoided.

Thyroid disorders and growth

The thyroid gland is to be found just beneath the Adam's apple (actually called the thyroid cartilage). It is an endocrine gland and, as such, produces a number of thyroid hormones, principally thyroxine (T4) and tri-iodothyronine (T3), both of which govern the rate of body metabolism. Overactivity of the gland leads to overactive cells, the increased consumption of energy and loss of weight as reserves are 'burnt-up'. Conversely, an underactive gland will lead all the biochemical reactions and processes in the body to slow down; the result will be less call on energy sources, and weight gain. Thyroid hormones are also essential for normal growth, and deficiency will lead to short stature. Brain nerve cells are reliant on thyroid hormones for normal activity, so mental deficiency can result from underactivity of the gland.

Neonatal thyroid abnormalities are very rare in Down's syndrome. In one study 12 out of 1,130 patients had thyroid dysfunction, but in four of these it was transient; the remainder had primary hypothyroidism, which should be identified by neonatal screening programmes. Persistent hypotonia (head, trunk and limbs), good weight gain despite very poor feeding, prolonged jaundice, dry skin, sparse hair and a hoarse cry are all signs of this disorder. Some of these symptoms overlap with the characteristics of Down's syndrome, and when doubt exists blood should be taken for thyroid function tests.

The main advent of thyroid disfunction is in the teenage years. In one study from Glasgow four out of 116 children were found to have thyroid disease; three were hypothyroid and one was hyperthyroid. About a third of them were found to have thyroid autoantibodies, and this has been reported in other studies. The matter needs further evaluation, but it would seem sensible to screen children with Down's syndrome with thyroid function tests, and for the presence of thyroid autoantibodies at about the age of 10, and then at intervals thereafter depending on the results of these investigations. It is not yet known what percentage of children with thyroid autoantibodies proceed to develop functional thyroid disorders and in what percentage it is merely a transient phenomenon.

Unnoticed hypothyroidism was found in one study to have

an adverse effect on intellectual performance. Pueschel, from Rhode Island Hospital, USA, has written extensively on Down's syndrome. He studied 151 young people with Down's syndrome and showed there was an increasing tendency with age for thyroid stimulating hormone (TSH) levels to rise as thyroxine (T4) levels fell. He compared the IQ of those with abnormal TSH and T4 to those with increased TSH alone, and to those with normal thyroid function tests. The results were 41.77, 53.8 and 55.3 respectively. Although Koch in 1965, in a double-blind study, found no benefit from the random administration of thyroxine, these data from Pueschel make a case for regular screening and appropriate treatment.

However, in a study carried out in the author's department thyroid function tests were performed on 122 children with Down's syndrome aged six to 14 years. One hundred and three adolescents (85 per cent of the group of 122) were resampled after an interval of 4–6 years when they were aged 10–20 years (median 14.4 years). Twenty of these young people had Isolated Raised TSH (with otherwise normal thyroid function) on initial testing. Fourteen (70 per cent) of these 20 were normal on second testing, and four (5 per cent) of the 83 with initial normal results had Isolated Raised TSH on second testing. Seventeen of 21 with Isolated Raised TSH had a thyrotrophin releasing hormone test within three months of first testing. The TSH result had become normal within three months in eight of these children. There was no association between reported clinical symptoms and Isolated Raised TSH but there were clear symptoms in two of the three with definite hypothyroidism. The likelihood of an abnormal result on second testing was 20 times higher when raised TSH and positive antibody status were present on first testing. This suggests that these results could be used as a basis to select a sub-group for further testing at, say, five-yearly intervals unless new symptoms emerge in the interim. The case for continuing to screen all those with Down's syndrome for hypothyroidism after initial testing is not supported by these results, but clearly further evaluation is required.

Growth retardation is a feature of Down's syndrome, and data exist on growth in 730 children, based on 4,650 observations up to the age of 18 years to allow assessment of growth in children with the syndrome. Another endocrine gland, the pituitary, which lies just below and has close connections with the fore-brain, is responsible for the production of a number of growth factors. These include human growth hormone and the somatomedins. They, like insulin, encourage cells to take up energy sources such as glucose from the blood and have an anabolic (building-up) effect on body metabolism.

Children with Down's syndrome show a deficiency in serum insulin-like growth factor (IGF-1). This growth-hormone-dependent somatomedin fails to rise during childhood and remains at a low concentration throughout life. The serum concentration of insulin-like growth factor 2 (IGF-2) in Down's syndrome is normal, and somatomedin and insulin receptors are also normal. A number of children have been described who have shown abnormalities of growth over and above that expected in a population of children with Down's syndrome. These children have responded to treatment with human growth hormone. The decision to treat, however, is not straightforward; growth hormone treatment increases the risk of leukaemia (see page 68), and the reason for treatment should always be well defined and understood from the child's point of view. There is no evidence that growth hormone increases learning ability.

Gonadotrophins (the sex hormones) will be reviewed in Chapter 9. From that discussion, and from data on thyroid and growth hormone function, it can be deduced that the biological activity of these hormones may be reduced. Although testicular failure in some males is primary, and auto-immune thyroiditis is an important cause of hypothyroidism, other factors are probably important. The research is yet to be done, but it is likely that target-organ failure plays a role in endocrine hypofunction. In target-organ failure there is adequate hormonal production but the 'target tissues' on which the hormones usually act fail to respond. The common factor may well be a disorder of membrane metabolism.

Skeletal abnormalities

Skull and middle-ear shape, and the possible effect on hearing, have already been considered. Absence of the 12th rib, incomplete fusion of the lower spinal vertebral arches, and fusion of the second and third toes are well described associations with Down's syndrome.

The top two bones in the spinal column, the atlas and the axis, have received a lot of attention. The spinal column is really a stack of bones, called vertebrae, which stand on top of each other. There is a hole down the middle of each, through which passes the spinal cord – a long cylinder containing millions of nerve cells transmitting messages for motor activity from the brain to muscles in the arms, legs and trunk, and gathering sensory information on pain, temperature, joint position and so on, and sending it back up to the brain. The atlas and the axis vertebrae, at the top of the spinal column, are very different in shape. The atlas supports the base of the skull above it, and its saucer shape allows nodding movement of the skull. The atlas has a large hole in its centre, through which part of the axis, the odontoid peg, protrudes; this allows pivoting side-to-side movement. All these vertebrae are joined by ligaments and muscles, but in Down's syndrome the ligaments tend to be lax and the muscle tone tends to be poor. This allows undue movement between the atlas and axis, and raises the danger of the odontoid peg squashing the spinal cord which lies just behind it.

This movement of the atlas on the axis is referred to as atlanto-axial dislocation, or subluxation. At one time the Department of Health issued guidance on children with Down's syndrome likely to undertake physical activity which might put them at increased risk of subluxation. This includes the hyperextension of the neck which occurs during the induction of anaesthesia, when a tube is passed into the wind-pipe.

Hospital-based studies indicate that there is undue movement of the odontoid peg relative to the atlas (4.5 mm or more) in up to 20 per cent of people with Down's syndrome, with a certain improvement as children get older. In the author's department clinical signs and symptoms that might predict atlanto-axial subluxation were studied prospectively in 135 of 180 children with Down's syndrome aged 6–14 years. X-rays of the cervical spine were taken in flexed, extended and neutral positions, and the percentage of abnormalities in each view was 14, 10 and 10 per cent respectively. If a child had an abnormal gait then the risk of having an abnormal neck X-ray was 2.91 times higher than if the gait was normal. Although 81 per cent of those with an abnormal gait had an abnormal X-ray, only 50 per cent of those with an abnormal X-ray had an abnormal gait. Nineteen children had repeat radiographs to assess the reliability of radiological diagnosis. Six had abnormalities; five of 19 (26 per cent) had an abnormality on the first X-ray and four of 19 (21 per cent) had an abnormality on a second radiograph, but only three (15 per cent) had an abnormality on both occasions in any view. We concluded that radiographs of the cervical spine are unreliable for identifying atlanto-axial subluxation in children with Down's syndrome, and we failed to identify any reliable clinical predictor.

It must be remembered that despite the frequency of the phenomenon, only 15 cases of spinal cord damage had been described in the 22-year period up to 1987.

In the author's opinion, given that X-rays of the neck are unreliable in showing instability, and given the very small risk involved, it is probably not worth screening children with Down's syndrome in this way. Common sense should apply, and anaesthetists be appraised of the risks of anaesthesia and parents appraised of the risks their children run when pursuing more active sports such as trampolining and high-diving.

This is now the basis of current Department of Health guidance. It is no longer a requirement to screen for atlanto-axial instability, and many young people with Down's syndrome who were previously excluded from sporting events can now enjoy the benefit of participation.

Gastrointestinal abnormalities

Constipation is a common symptom in Down's syndrome. Poor muscle tone, mobility and fluid intake probably all contribute, especially in young babies. The symptom tends to improve, as all these things improve, with age. Attention should be paid to an adequate fluid intake and amount of roughage in the diet.

Babies may be helped to open their bowels by gently inserting a cotton-bud coated with petroleum jelly a short distance into the anus (back passage). For older children, if the bowels have not opened for, say, three days, a glycerine suppository usually helps. If the difficulty persists, the family doctor may wish to prescribe medication that keeps the stools soft or laxatives.

Developmental abnormalities of the intestines are rare in Down's syndrome but are most likely to present in the newborn period. Duodenal atresia is the commonest. The duodenum is the first part of the folded tube-like structure known as the intestine. The intestines begin at the stomach and end at the anus; their job is to break down and absorb food, a process called digestion. Atresia means the tube has failed to canalise properly so that the stomach is passing its contents on into a blind-ending cul-de-sac.

Duodenal atresia presents with vomiting (as there is a build-up of milk) and absolute constipation (as no food can pass the blockage). Unlike other forms of intestinal obstruction, there is no abdominal distension as the blockage is at the beginning of the bowel, which cannot therefore become distended with gas. There may or may not be bilious vomiting, depending on whether the atresia has arisen before or after the bile duct enters the duodenum. There is often a history of polyhydramnios (more fluid than usual around the growing baby in the amniotic sac in pregnancy) because the normal flow of amniotic fluid through the baby's intestines has been disrupted. A plain abdominal X-ray reveals the characteristic 'double bubble' of gas in the stomach and first part of the duodenum. After initial resuscitation, corrective surgery can be carried out.

Malabsorption (poor absorption of nutrients from the intestine) is now recognised as a problem in some people with Down's syndrome. Recently there have been reports of an increased incidence of coeliac disease. This is an immune-mediated disorder in which an allergy is developed to the gliadin fraction of gluten in wheatgerm. The intestinal mucosa becomes inflamed and then atrophies (undergoes a significant degree of shrinkage). The absorptive surface is then reduced, and malabsorption results. Treatment is with a gluten-free diet that leads to recovery of the mucosal surface of the bowel.

Specific malabsorption of vitamin B12 has also been reported in a three-year-old girl with Down's syndrome. She presented with loss of weight, diarrhoea, day-time wetting, cold peripheries, lethargy, loss of appetite and a rash. A peripheral blood count showed the large red cells (macrocytosis) typical of B12 deficiency, and a Schilling test confirmed that this was due to malabsorption. Unlike other reported cases, she did not have protein in her urine. She made a good recovery with B12 injections. There have been no other reported cases so far, and this one may never be repeated, but it does serve to emphasise the importance of not attributing all symptomatology to the syndrome itself.

Disordered immunity/leukaemia

People with Down's syndrome have poorly functioning immune systems; they have relatively poor responses to infections and tend to mount inappropriate attacks on their own bodies. This is a very active area of research, and this section will highlight some of the important developments.

One of the most important components of human immunity are the T-cell lymphocytes, so-called because they are produced in the thymus gland, which is found in the upper part of the chest. It is their job to recognise invading substances as 'not-self', in which case they multiply rapidly to form clones of cells that neutralise the invader.

It is suggested that there is an intrinsic T-cell immune defect in Down's syndrome which is responsible for the increased susceptibility to malignancy, infection and auto-immune disorders (see above under thyroid function). In the laboratory T cells can be made to multiply in a non-specific way with the use of a substance called phytohaemagglutinin (PHA). In Down's syndrome the level of T cells appears to be normal for the first 10 years of life and then declines. More specific reactions can be studied with the use of monoclonal antibodies (very specific invading proteins) such as anti-CD3. The response of lymphocytes in Down's syndrome in this situation is significantly reduced at any age. Studies have shown that this is not due to the T cells being unable to latch on to (bind to) the foreign protein, nor to defective interaction with monocytes which 'mop-up the debris'. Instead, overexpanded populations of specialised T cells which limit and confine the immune response have been found. These are called suppressor and natural killer cells. The problem may then be due to excess numbers (another gene dose effect) of inhibitory immunoregulatory cells.

One can speculate that the inefficient response may also be due to the abnormalities of membrane function. The T lymphocytes of younger people with Down's syndrome have significantly elevated levels of cyclic guanine monophosphate, a substance which acts as a substrate for an enzyme called guanylate cyclase, which in turn is very important for normal membrane and cell wall function. In this respect they resemble cells of older people without Down's syndrome and the immunodeficient state that accompanies ageing.

Lymphocyte functional antigen-1 (LFA-1) assists the binding of immune lymphocytes to antigens. A large part of this substance is coded for at 21q22. Again, because of the gene-dosage effect, LFA-1 is seen in increased levels on Down's syndrome cells. This leads the lymphocytes to show increased adhesiveness, with resulting non-specific binding. The immune response therefore lacks a degree of specificity, and becomes inefficient.

The cell surface receptor for an important substance called interferon, produced against viruses, is coded for on chromosome 21. This leads sensitivity to the anti-viral effects of interferon to be several-fold greater in Down's syndrome, even though interferon production is the same. It is possible that people with Down's syndrome are more susceptible to viral infection because this sensitivity of the interferon receptors to the immunosuppressive effects of interferon leads to a premature shutdown of the response.

There are a number of conditions with an autoimmune basis that present in people with Down's syndrome. Thyroid disease has already been mentioned; type 1 (insulin-dependent) diabetes is another example. Additionally, vitiligo (patchy loss of skin coloration), where lymphocytes attack the melanocytes in the skin (which produce pigment), and alopoecia areata (hair loss, mentioned earlier) may also be seen in excess. Coeliac disease also appears to be more common in Down's syndrome (see page 67).

The thymus gland, where the T cells are produced, has a different structure in many young people with Down's syndrome. There are altered lymphocyte sub-populations in the peripheral blood and thymus, with evidence of T-cell activation and premature ageing so that T-cell subsets are different from those in the general population. The tendency to autoimmune conditions may be associated with the fact that the HLA alleles, which confer genetic susceptibility to autoimmunity, are more prevalent in Down's syndrome.

The onset of diabetes in children who also have Down's syndrome tends to be earlier than in those children in the general population. This could be explained by an autoimmune process starting much earlier in childhood (the bio-chemical predisposition to diabetes in Down's syndrome related to phospho-fructo-kinase activity has already been mentioned). Studies suggest that children with diabetes and Down's syndrome also have a different HLA profile to those in the general population, but this needs to be confirmed with further study.

To date there is no evidence that gene over-expression (given that three copies of chromosome 21 are present instead of two) is linked to the appearance of autoimmunity. However, there are several ways in which the extra copy of chromosome 21 could increase a tendency to autoimmunity, and further research is looking closely into these possibilities. If two copies of one chromosome are inherited from one parent, as happens in Down's syndrome (plus the third copy from the other parent), this is called disomic homogeneity (see Chapter 2). A gene called AIRE (autoimmune regulator) is on chromosome 21, and its over-expression could lead to an inefficient immune response. Similarly, Amyloid Precursor Protein (APP), linked to the development of Alzheimer's disease (see page 73), could with overactivity of superoxide dismutase lead to the early ageing of immune cells, tissue destruction and increased tissue inflammation.

There is an important membrane protein called ICOS (or LICOS when bound) which switches lymphocytes on to deal with foreign invading protein. Activation leads to proliferation of T cells and cytokine production. It could be that the over-expression of LICOS (produced from a gene on chromosome 21) leads to increased lymphocyte damage and cytokine production, thereby making organ function more severe. Further studies are necessary.

This impairment of cell-mediated immune reactions probably leads to inefficient immunosurveillance (the T cells search and destroy any substance that is foreign, abnormal or 'not-self'). An increased susceptibility to infection tends not to be of great clinical importance after infancy, although increased numbers of skin and middle-ear infections are reported. One popular misconception is that people with Down's syndrome are at risk of contracting hepatitis B (the type contracted from blood products). This is not the case, although hepatitis A (infectious hepatitis) used to be quite prevalent in institutions, which is probably how the misunderstanding arose.

Although increased risk of infection is not of great practical importance, the 1 per cent reported incidence of leukaemia is 14–18-fold higher than in the general population. Interestingly, the Danish study that showed an 18-fold overall risk of leukaemia in Down's syndrome showed no cases over the age of 29 and a very specific risk of myeloid leukaemia. There was a decreased risk of other cancers in all age groups. Studies show that up to about 20 years ago children with Down's syndrome who had leukaemia were often not referred to specialist centres and were not getting standard treatment, and the results of treatment were significantly worse than those of children in the general population. Treatment management and outcome data are monitored in the United Kingdom by the UKCCSG (United Kingdom Childhood Cancer Study Group). Their data show that some children with Down's syndrome had a unique form of myeloid leukaemia known as megakaryoblastic leukaemia, which is very, very rare in other children. It is, however, quite sensitive to chemotherapy, with a high chance of cure. The initial remission rate in children with Down's syndrome is not quite so good as for other children (83 per cent versus 92 per cent), the difference largely being due to an increased risk of induction (at the start of treatment) deaths (17 per cent versus 4 per cent). However, intensive supportive treatment, including antibiotic treatment, in the initial period at a regional centre should serve to minimise these deaths. The overall five-year survival rate is virtually the same as for other children (59 per cent versus 60 per cent). Relapse risk is significantly less than for other children (8 per cent versus 39 per cent) and the risk of death in remission is significantly greater than for other children (21 per cent versus 8 per cent), probably because of the increased vulnerability to infection during intensive chemotherapy already mentioned.

The risk of acute lymphoblastic leukaemia is significantly higher in Down's syndrome, and most children tend to be aged two to nine years, with few seen before or after those ages. They tend to have common lymphoblastic leukaemia without adverse outcome genetic markers. When the results of UKALL X (conducted from 1985 to 1990) and UKALL XI (conducted from 1990 to 1997) were compared, important observations were made. For children with Down's syndrome the risk of death in the first remission fell from 21 per cent to 8 per cent (for other children from 4 to 2 per cent). The overall five-year survival was 73 per cent, which was significantly poorer than for other children (82 per cent), though in the later study (UKALL XI) it showed improvement. The event-free survival (that is staying free of a relapse or complications) was 53 per cent versus 63 per cent in other children, and the five-year relapse rate was 55 per cent for Down's syndrome and 34 per cent for other children. Again, the excess mortality rate seems to be due to supra-added infections seen more commonly in Down's syndrome. They tend to be fungal infections, which may lead to an alteration in policy so that anti-fungal agents are used earlier in the future. Looked at overall, the data clearly support early referral to a specialist centre of any child with leukaemia for the expert application of standardised treatment regimes.

As a well-reported but very rare condition in Down's syndrome, newborn babies may show a very raised white cell count and primitive bone marrow cells known as blasts cells in the peripheral blood. When the blood film is viewed the features are indistinguishable from these seen in acute myeloid leukaemia in childhood. In the vast majority of cases the baby remains well and the blood count abnormality resolves steadily. Very occasionally, small doses of cytotoxic drugs used in the treatment of leukaemia have to be administered. It is not known why this abnormality is more common in Down's syndrome. It is also not clear what percentage of babies who show this condition go on to develop leukaemia later in childhood, though this could be as many as one in five. Where this does occur, effective treatment is available.

Epilepsy

Epilepsy is more common in Down's syndrome than in the general population, but nevertheless remains relatively rare, affecting between 1 and 5 per cent. Those children who develop epilepsy tend to be the more severely intellectually impaired, but there are notable exceptions to this rule. As in all other children with epilepsy, the character of the seizure type must be defined by means of a detailed history, assessment and EEG (electroencephalographic) recordings. An EEG is performed with the child wearing a sort of 'crown' on the head for 10 to 15 minutes, the electrodes in the crown detecting electrical activity in the brain. The pattern of electrical activity allows the doctor to decide if there is any evidence of epilepsy and, if so, just what form it takes. From this information, advice on outlook and the most appropriate form of therapy can be given.

Some of the drugs used to treat epilepsy, like anti-cancer drugs, interfere with folate metabolism; because of this, long-term effects on the blood count and bone metabolism need to be monitored on an annual basis.

Ageing and Alzheimer's disease

Alzheimer's disease is the most common form of pre-senile dementia in Britain, affecting 5 per cent of the population over 65 and 20 per cent over the age of 80. It accounts for 50 per cent of those with dementia in the general population. Pathologists can diagnose the condition when they see specific appearances on brain biopsy; these are neuritic plaques and neurofibrillary tangles.

Particular neuronal systems are affected, involving the memory and cognitive systems found in a part of the brain called the hippocampus and its cortical connections. As this neuronal loss is selective, a problem involving specific neuro-transmitters can be ruled out, although a deficiency of cholinergic nerve cells has been demonstrated. The neuritic plaques have a core of protein mixed with aluminium silicates, dystrophic (abnormally grown) neurites and neuro-glia (cells that support nerve-cells in the brain). There is an association between aluminium and Alzheimer's disease, but there is no clear dose-related trend. The difference in bioavailability of aluminium from differing sources may be important, as may genetic susceptibility; more clinical and epidemiological studies are needed. The proteinaceous material in the core seems to be A4 or beta-amyloid. Chromosome 21 houses the amyloid precursor protein (APP) gene, one of the early-onset Alzheimer's disease genes. Malfunction of the APP gene causes abnormal processing of amyloid precursor protein. When amyloid precursor protein is processed abnormally, fragments of the protein, called beta-amyloid, begin to accumulate in the brain and form the amyloid plaques found between nerve cells. It may be that a gene dosage effect for this peptide is not causative but rather that the Alzheimer's disease locus lies close to that of A4-amyloid within band 21q21.

The disease is particularly common in Down's syndrome and increasingly so after the age of 40. Some authors have claimed that people with Down's syndrome inevitably develop the disease eventually, but others dispute this. Early manifestations are an insidious loss of memory and intellectual function, which lead to confusion, disorientation and ultimately to profound mental and physical disability.

The diagnosis is made by excluding other conditions that lead to confusional states and dementia. Magnetic-Resonance Imaging (MRI) scanning can be helpful in excluding other causes, although the appearances are very often non-specific, and multiple infarct dementia, so common in the elderly, is rare in Down's syndrome because of the rarity of atheroma (see Chapter 2). Positron emission tomography (PET) scanning reveals functional changes at a biochemical level, and in one study was shown to be more useful than MRI in terms of reflecting the degree of pathology. Study of neurotransmitters in cerebrospinal fluid gives non-specific results, and the electroencephalogram (EEG) is unhelpful. Clinical evaluation by a caring and astute physician remains the mainstay of investigation of people with learning difficulties who develop dementia.

Various attempts have been made at replacement therapy, concentrating particularly on the deficient cholinergic system. In addition to using the acetyl-choline precursors choline and lecithin, anticholinesterases and receptor agonists have been used. Anticholinesterases boost the naturally occurring levels of acetyl-choline, while agonists boost its effect. Trials had not shown any important benefits until 1986, when Summers reported significant improvement in some patients with the use of tetra-hydro-aminoacridine (THA). THA is a potent centrally acting anticholinesterase and stimulant; it increases the need for free choline, and in some trials it has been given with lecithin. As with all anticholinergics, it can give unwanted gastrointestinal effects and hypotension. More seriously, in up to a third of people it can cause hepatotoxicity (liver damage) due to a chronic hepatitis. This is said to be reversible on stopping the drug, but further evaluation of its risks and benefits are needed.

Meanwhile a pragmatic approach to therapy has to be adopted. The major tranquillisers can bring calmness to the very disturbed, but side-effects may be troublesome. More importantly, a close liaison needs to be established between learning difficulty support services who comfort those affected and their families. Research continues into the causes and treatment of this common disorder.

7

Going to school

Young children with Down's syndrome who have been taught and encouraged from their earliest days benefit from attending a local playgroup or nursery school before going on into the full-time educational system. They should also enjoy the activities undertaken by other children of the same age, such as ballet classes, swimming and horseriding. However, it is often the search for an appropriate nursery placement that first brings parents into contact with their local education authority (LEA).

The LEA and statements of special educational need

The 1981 Education Act was an important step towards ensuring a right to integration in mainstream education for children with special needs. The Act also established the duty of education authorities to identify those children for whom it was necessary to make a statement and to assess what help was needed for each child.

The 1993 Education Act built on these foundations and instituted the Special Educational Needs Tribunal, a body independent from the LEAs to which parents may appeal against certain decisions of the LEA. The current law setting out the duties and responsibilities of LEAs, Governors and schools to pupils with special educational needs is now set out in the Education Act 1996 as amended by the School Standards and Framework Act 1998 and the Special Educational Needs and Disability Act 2001. The details follow.

First an officer of the Local Education Authority (LEA) carries out a formal assessment to assess a child's strengths and weaknesses. They are required to seek advice from a number of professional sources as well as from the parent. A statement of special educational needs is then drawn up identifying the needs of the child and specifying the special educational provision to meet those needs. Provision for nursery nurses or non-teaching assistants is commonly made, to supervise the activity of children with learning difficulties in the classroom and at breaktime, along with the provision of appropriate remedial therapy such as speech therapy. Unless the parent makes suitable arrangements themselves, the LEA has a legal duty to arrange that the special educational provision set out in the statement is made for the child.

The law requires the LEA to educate children with special needs in mainstream school unless the parent does not want this or to do so would be incompatible with the provision of efficient education for other children. The LEA cannot refuse the child a mainstream place if reasonable steps taken by it or the school would allow inclusion without detracting from the efficient education of the other children. If the child is refused the preferred mainstream school because of unsuitability or an inefficient use of resources, the LEA must offer him or her a place at another mainstream school. Low ability, limited speech or the cost of special educational provision are not lawful reasons for denying a mainstream place altogether.

Parents may ask for an assessment of their child at any stage. Before their child is two years old, if it is necessary for their special educational provision to be decided by the LEA, the LEA may make an assessment with the consent of the parent – and is duty bound to do so at the parents' request. Such assessment and any statement made are not subject to the formal process that the law requires when the child is over two.

The LEA may learn of a child's special educational needs from their doctor, who has a duty to tell the parent and then the education authority of any child under five who has (or probably has) special educational needs.

After the age of two the LEA has a duty to identify those children with special needs whose special educational provision they need to decide. The LEA must notify parents if they propose to assess their child and give parents 29 days in which to comment. If parents request an assessment for a child over two, the LEA must comply if it is necessary to make an assessment and there has not been one in the past six months. If the LEA refuses to assess following such a request, the parent may appeal to the Special Educational Needs & Disability Tribunal.

Parents must receive notice of any examination of their child for the purpose of the assessment and have a right to be present. Parents who refuse to take their child for an assessment or examination without a reasonable excuse commit an offence and can be prosecuted and fined.

The assessment must generally be completed within ten weeks of the LEA's decision to make an assessment. Within a further two weeks the LEA must either notify the parent of their decision not to make a statement and the parent's right to appeal to the Special Educational Tribunal against this decision or send to the parent a copy of the proposed statement.

The proposed statement will be in the same form and with the same contents as the LEA plan to put into the final statement except that Part 4 will be blank instead of naming the school the child is to attend. Parents then have an opportunity to let the LEA know their views on the contents of the statement and express a preference for the school they want for their child. Parents' views (known as representations) and the name of their preferred school must be sent to the LEA within 15 days of receiving the statement unless the parents exercise their right to request a meeting with an officer to discuss the statement. If a meeting is called and parents are still unhappy, they can request a further meeting to discuss any of the professional advice with an appropriate person. Where parents request a meeting, the 15 days within which to make representations or express a preference for a school runs from the date of the meeting or the further meeting if one is requested. The final statement should be made within eight weeks of sending the proposed statement. Parents can appeal to the Special Educational Needs Tribunal against the contents of the final statement, including the school named. All appeals to the Special Educational Needs Tribunal must be made within two months of the LEA notifying the parents of their right to appeal.

After statements are made they must be reviewed within 12 months. Different rules apply to the first annual review following the child's 14th birthday, which begins to plan for the child's adult life by drawing up a transition plan.

The recent educational climate has caused some concern to parents of children with special educational needs. The baseline of the national curriculum will not be obtainable by all children with Down's syndrome. There is anxiety that mainstream schools will be less inclined to accommodate children with special educational needs because of their likely effect on school league tables. Special educational provision for children with Down's syndrome can be expensive, and with schools holding their own budget they may see such children as a charge on their resources, particularly where the statement is not sufficiently specific to commit the LEA to any expenditure.

The year 2001 brought changes to the way schools were funded for the support of children with special educational needs. Previously the LEA held a central budget and employed a group of peripatetic teachers who generally visited a number of schools, assessing and supporting a number of children and the teachers and support staff they were involved with. The central funding along with the central pool of teachers allowed them to develop an *esprit de corps*, to offer each other professional support, to share experience and develop skills. Now that the budget is devolved there is the potential for the service to become more fragmented. Teachers may work in one or two schools and rarely come together as a group. Professional isolation could lead to them become deskilled. It is important that systems for continuing professional development are put in place and maintained. The Down's Syndrome Association opposed this change and will be watching the situation carefully.

A school's attitude to special education can be considerably influenced by the governing body. Governors have a duty to do their best to secure special educational provision for children with learning difficulties in their schools. With this in mind it is clearly of advantage to parents of children with Down's syndrome to get themselves elected to the governing bodies of schools.

Many officers of LEAs, educational authorities and head-teachers are very sympathetic to and supportive of the ideal of integration.

When parents are first thinking about finding a playschool or school for their children, they are well advised to visit as many establishments as possible in the area. The final choice is often a difficult one, and in the end is based on a mixture of factors including the previous experience a school has of children with special needs, perceived attitude of the staff and geographical location. At times parents will feel hurt when they come up against headteachers who seem to lack understanding, but persistence coupled with the philosophy behind the Education Act and the goodwill of most professionals will usually secure success in the end.

SUMMARY OF PROCEDURES

Children under two

- Parent can ask for assessment.
- District Health Authority must tell parent, then Educational Authority, that child may have special educational needs.
- Education Authority may (with consent of parent) and must (at request of parent) make an assessment, which can be of any kind and may result in a Statement of Special Educational Needs.

Children between two and 19

- Authorities have a duty to identify children whose special educational needs make it necessary for the authority to decide on special educational provision.
- Parents can request assessment and authorities cannot unreasonably refuse.
- Parents can appeal against refusal to assess.

Assessment

- Notice to parents – 29 days to comment.
- If authority decides not to assess, must notify parent.
- Parents must receive notices of any examinations; have a right to be present and to submit information.
- Parents who fail to see that their children turn up for examinations without reasonable excuse may be guilty of offence and fined.

After assessment

- Authority may decide not to make statement, may issue a Note in Lieu of a Statement instead.
- Must inform parents of right of appeal to SEN Tribunal.
- If authority decides to make statement, must serve copy of

proposed statement on parents and enable parents to state a preference for a school.
- Parents have 15 days in which to express a preference and make representations or ask for meeting with officer, and a further 15 days to ask for other meetings with professionals to discuss professional advice provided to authority (which must be given to parents as part of statement).
- Authority, after considering parents' views, can make statement in the same or changed form (but must include name of school in statement) or decide not to make it; must inform parents.
- If statement is made, must be sent to parents with notice of right to appeal in writing to SEN Tribunal, which can confirm statement, or ask LEA to reconsider it.

After statement is made
- Statements must be reviewed within every 12 months.
- Young people aged 14+ must have a Transition Plan drawn up after each Annual Review.
- Parents can appeal if the statement is amended or if there is a decision to cease to maintain the statement, or a refusal to name a different school.
- The LEA must see that special educational provision set out in statement is made.

Liaison

One of the keys to a child's success and happiness is that parents, therapists, carers and staff in the school or in clinics liaise with each other so that aims and achievements can be coordinated as much as possible. In this respect parents have a key role, but they often appreciate the support and advocacy of one of the pre-school support team members in establishing links with education, health or social services.

If parents have been encouraging their child since birth through natural play guided by therapists, they will want to continue this process by reinforcing the activities that are taught at playschool, and later at primary school. Children with Down's syndrome will often not be able to report clearly what they experience at school and this makes close liaison essential, especially if remedial therapists are involved; regular discussions of a child's developments and achievements at home and at school are often enlightening for parents and staff alike. Communication logs, daily diaries or home/school books can be helpful in this respect, in which both parents and teachers may keep a record of significant events.

Some parents may feel apprehensive about contacting 'professionals' in this way, or even about asking teachers and nursery school staff to take their child in the first place. Some may expect a more structured teaching programme than is actually provided. In all these cases it is important for contact to be made with the relevant people. Invariably staff will be more than willing to meet the needs of each child and family.

On a more practical level, if the child has a heart defect it is important that everyone is made aware of this and of the limitations it may place on activity. A school nurse should be involved, and contact between the school, hospital and community paediatricians, and the family doctor are particularly helpful. In general, though, activity should be limited as little as possible so as to increase independence, confidence and a sense of belonging.

If school staff have only a broad knowledge of Down's syndrome, they may feel that the list of physical needs is rather daunting. They need to be made aware that not all children with Down's syndrome have all the problems at once, if at all. Many children will already have learned to cope with any problems in their own way by the time they get to school age. Staff should be prepared to learn from the child, which will offer obvious benefits. In the classroom the Down's syndrome becomes irrelevant. Each child's individual strengths and weaknesses need assessment.

Finally it should be remembered that a move from the relative shelter of home to nursery school or playschool, or from nursery school to infant school and then to primary school, can be a big step for any child. Parents should, if possible, visit the school on a number of occasions with the child, so as to give them a chance to look around and help them feel comfortable with their new environment.

Preparation

While it is obviously helpful for the staff at playschool or school if a child can recognise their own peg, and cope with dressing, undressing, toileting and so on, these are not skills that are necessary to start with. Overemphasis on this sort of

CLOSE Visit Notes — Mon 5th Nov

During the course of this visit I played 2 group games with Michael as follows;

Find it

Perception Lotto. - Each child has a picture & then has to find smaller picture cards within their picture. Michael enjoyed this and tried very hard to find the pictures. (He had a house). He found the larger items e.g. bicycle easy and the smaller pictures more difficult e.g. goldfish bowl. This was no different to the problems experienced by all the children I played this with.

Coloured Cube Designs

This consisted of cube designs and wooden cubes to copy the designs with. Once again, like the other children Michael found it relatively easy to place the cubes in the correct places on the cards but, extremely difficult to copy the design below the card.

When I left Michael was absorbed in completing quite a complicated inset puzzle.

I will run a Makaton session next Mon lunchtime.

J. Gracie.

Sample of note written by one of the teachers in a complex learning difficulties support service for parents at home.

issue can lead to anxiety in children and their parents. Children learn quickly from other children; children with Down's syndrome often find copying very easy and are likely to pick up what is required of them quite quickly. However, a few practical hints that may be of use are:

- Garments should be labelled with the child's name to help easy identification in busy cloakrooms.

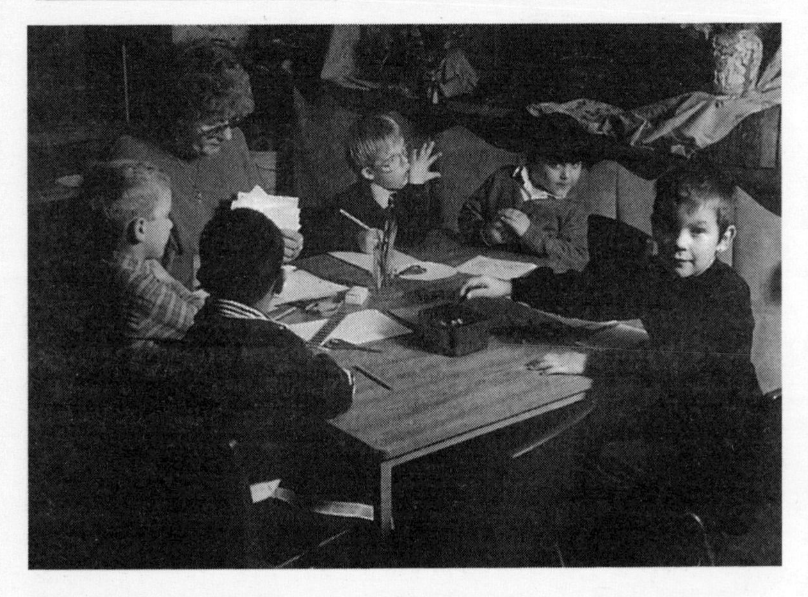

In the classroom: small group working with classroom helper, offering benefit to all class members.

- Clothes can be trendy but not 'best', as they are liable to get paint splashed on them, or pulled during boisterous play.
- Clothes that are easy to remove for going to the toilet are advisable – avoid dungarees with complicated fastenings.
- Ski-pants or track-suit bottoms allow a child to crawl around on cold floors without getting scuffed knees and cold legs.
- Tops should have sleeves that can be pushed up the arms easily, with no cuff bottoms. This allows paint and water play without the child getting soaked.
- Long hair should be tied back, partly to keep it out of the way, but also to discourage other children from playing with their new friend like a doll.

It is important to introduce children to their new nursery staff or teachers. They are bound to be apprehensive about being left to start with. Parents are often allowed to stay a short time in the introductory days, and it can be helpful to leave a familiar object for comfort.

As the child's concept of time is poor, it helps if teachers explain that the child's mother and father will be coming back after a certain activity or event, for example 'When lunch is ready', 'After lunch', 'After you have made a picture'. The description should be accurate, and the teacher should ensure that what has been described really is the last activity or event of the school day. Children with Down's syndrome often understand instructions literally, and if a parent is supposed to be arriving after a child 'has made a picture' and the day's events are not programmed, the child may do nothing more once the picture is finished and remain rather confused about why it is not time to go home.

Social skills

The ability range in Down's syndrome, although lower and generally slower, is as wide as in any other group of children. It always bears repeating that facial appearance gives no indication of the individual child's ability or potential. It is worth emphasising that a child's personality is determined by their home and family background as much as by their chromosomal make-up.

A popular misconception is that children with Down's syndrome are always lovable and affectionate. Some are, but only some of the time. All children can be annoying at times, behave badly and be disobedient or easily distracted; children with Down's syndrome are no exception. However, children with Down's syndrome can get into difficulties in their efforts to help or be friendly; for example they may greet people in an inappropriate way, by kissing or hugging. This tendency gets better as social rules are learnt through observing the behaviour of other children. Adults should treat a child with Down's syndrome as they would all other members of the class or group. Classmates, too, need to be encouraged to interact normally both in and out of school; there is often a tendency to 'mother', as the child with Down's syndrome is seen to be vulnerable. Children at school age are very sensitive to other children's ability, and naturally feel protective and supportive if they sense a child is less able than they are. If the reaction of others is appropriate, children with Down's syndrome will learn confidence, encouragement and independence.

Behaviour

Staff at playschool or school may have no previous experience of Down's syndrome but just the same misconceptions as held by the parents at the time of the child's birth. It is therefore helpful if parents paint a picture of their child for the teachers in the reception class, as misunderstandings are far easier to prevent than to undo.

Many children with Down's syndrome have long memories, particularly for events and people, which leads them to be routine conscious and quite resistant to change. This leads them to be easily upset if explained plans or the usual routine is unexpectedly changed. Whenever possible, changes in staffing or activity that can be foreseen should be explained and presented in a positive manner. Children with Down's syndrome are often described as being stubborn. In fact they can often become very engrossed in the simplest of tasks, putting on socks or drawing a picture, and when asked to perform a different activity display temporary frustration. Confrontation is best avoided, and if simple explanation does not work then imaginative distraction is called for; an attempt to make them laugh often works.

Stages of development usually last longer in any child with learning difficulties. This means that irritating habits may take more than the expected time to be extinguished. Sometimes children with Down's syndrome go through a stage when they repeat what is said to them in an effort to please rather than because what they are saying is true. They may answer 'Yes' when they actually mean 'No', with the correct answer probably following on after a brief pause.

A strong sense of humour and a mischievous streak are often features of children with Down's syndrome. This love of mischief, if combined with boredom, can lead to inconvenient attention-seeking behaviour, like hiding the car keys or father's wallet. As with all young children, it is advisable to keep an eye on an unoccupied child with Down's syndrome, particularly if they are extraordinarily quiet.

Discipline and the teaching of structure and limits play a key role for a slow learner. A child with Down's syndrome who is not taught to behave is effectively given an additional disadvantage. As with any child in a new environment, after a period of assessment a child with Down's syndrome is likely to 'test' the adults in charge of them. A firm but sympathetic, patient response is required. It must be remembered that boredom is a common cause for frequent bad behaviour; it is important to ensure that the work set for the child is adequately stimulating and not underestimating of ability.

To encourage any undesirable behaviour by laughter or smiles when the child is young may lead to later problems that are not so easy to sort out. It is far more important to praise good behaviour frequently than to give attention to misbehaviour. Misbehaviour should be stopped with the minumum of fuss, or even ignored. Criticism and the emphasis of failure merely undermine confidence. These twin strategies – the praising of good behaviour and the ignoring of bad behaviour – are something that should evolve through discussions between parents and teaching staff; inconsistency leaves children confused and poorly behaved.

Hearing and sight

As explained in Chapter 6, many children with Down's syndrome are prone to colds, and the resultant catarrh can invade the Eustachian tube (leading from the throat to the middle ear) and temporarily affect hearing. If parents or staff suspect such a hearing loss, a full assessment should be obtained. Hearing loss may make learning even more difficult and delay the development of language concepts.

If a child has to wear a hearing aid they will undoubtedly need help with it at school, and this ought to be explained to the staff. It ought also to be explained that the use of the hearing aid may give rise to a fear or dislike of loud noise.

Many children with Down's syndrome need to wear glasses, and these should be chosen to suit the child's individual facial features. One aspect of Down's syndrome is a small bridge to the nose, which means that glasses tend to slip down and become a nuisance rather than useful. Frames less likely to slip are available, with a different bridge and longer ear pieces. Contact lenses are a successful alternative in many, but need careful supervision.

Teachers should check that the child arrives each day with the glasses and departs with them at the end of each session.

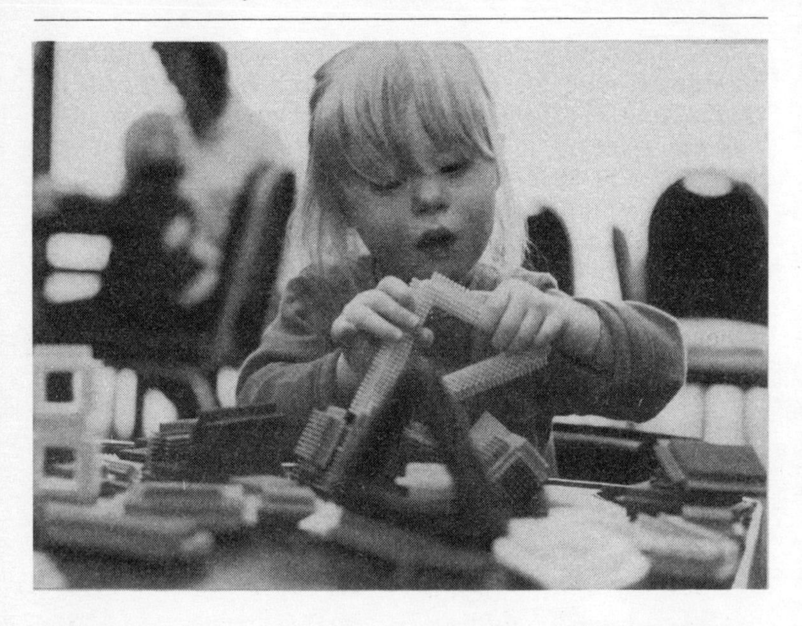

Children with Down's syndrome enjoy the same activities as others.

Teachers need to know if a child needs assistance in using the glasses and whether they need to be used all the time or only for close work. The glasses should also be checked after meals to see if they need cleaning.

The eyes of a child with Down's syndrome may not adapt quickly from bright light to shadow. This can cause the child to trip on unseen steps or uneven floors. Staff should be aware that a child with poor sight should be allowed to hold a book wherever is found to be most convenient, even if it is rather close to the eyes or tilted.

Finally, if a child is sight or hearing impaired, they will need to be able to see their teacher's face. A central position near the front is ideal, avoiding being placed facing a window or any other bright source of light.

Physical activities and health

As explained earlier, children with Down's syndrome have lower muscle tone than other children, and this can give rise to problems with coordination and gait. In particular, slack hip muscles can mean that physical activity is difficult. Because of this, extra encouragement and help may be needed for the child to achieve exercises involving hopping, skipping, running, climbing, kicking and balancing. This may give rise to frustration in team games and sport at times, but the children should never be discouraged from joining in. Other children tend to be good coaches, and swimming, dancing, PE and games will all help with muscle tone, general fitness and coordination. Participation should always be encouraged and achievement praised.

At meal times it should be remembered that a child with Down's syndrome often has an excellent appetite but may be prone to excess weight gain. Obesity can cause serious problems. Kind dinner-ladies have been known to get great delight from seeing third helpings disappear with immense voracity, but they need appropriate advice. A good diet is to be encouraged, in addition to exercise, and refined sugars avoided in sweets and drinks.

Poor coordination of the muscles of chewing and swallowing may cause a child with Down's syndrome to eat slowly. This needs bringing to the attention of the staff, so that extra time can be allowed and food chewed properly.

At break-time in cold weather, children with Down's syndrome often need slightly more attention than usual (advice to put on or take off a pullover or coat) because of their poor temperature control and vulnerable skin.

With appropriate preparation, attending nursery, and later school, is an enjoyable experience for all children with Down's syndrome. They have their first taste of social independence and have many new learning experiences. Parents see their toddlers emerging as young children ready to take the next important and exciting developmental steps.

8

Progress at school

Children with Down's syndrome learn best from a combination of visual, practical and spoken styles of teaching rather than purely spoken instruction, and progress consistently when emphasis is placed on praise and confidence building. Rewarding achievement with simple stars or tick charts can be very effective motivation. Where reward systems are in place at home to encourage a particular developmental step such as toilet training it is entirely appropriate to use the same system in school. It can be most effective to share some goals and strategies both at home and at school, while remembering that a regular and normal home life should take precedence over perpetual, formal teaching at home.

All of us respond to praise and it is worth remembering to speak only good of a child when in earshot; children will want to live up to the expectations of the adults they like, and will understand much more of what is being said around them than adults will usually give them credit for. Positive terminology, such as 'learning difficulty' or even 'special needs', is preferable to negative terms such as 'handicapped'.

Good communication between home and school is very important. Nothing beats face to face personal contact, but a home/school diary can help parents to reinforce learning taking place in school and help teachers to know what the child has been doing at home at weekends and during holidays. This is particularly useful for children with spoken language delay and can enable them to take part in story time and carpet time activities as well as sharing news and establishing the child's areas of interest for project and literacy work. By following up what is happening in school, parents can help children practise and reinforce new skills. A home/school book should be monitored to ensure that it remains a positive form of communication and does not simply turn into a list of complaints by staff or parents.

Differences in school-based 'academic' ability between children with Down's syndrome and their averagely developing peers will become more apparent as children progress through school. Children who learn at a slower rate than the norm are still making individual progress and need to be rewarded and praised for the steps that they make. As children get older it will become increasingly necessary to differentiate the teaching materials to make schoolwork meaningful and appropriate to the child's individual progress and ability. Children should have access to a broad and balanced curriculum and have the opportunity to take part in all subject areas of the national curriculum.

Every encouragement and opportunity for a child to make individual progress should be given. Some things to consider may be:

- Children with Down's syndrome do not always instigate the learning process. The class teacher should identify which step the child needs to learn next.
- It may help to simplify spoken instruction so that a child can gradually learn to repeat as accompaniment to their actions; for example 'Hold, over and push through' for doing up buttons.
- One should not assume that the child will understand language used in a new context. With terms such as 'top of the page', 'first', 'last', 'a lot' and 'more' (in the mathematical sense), a child's comprehension may lead to a very literal interpretation.

Learning practical tasks can be greatly assisted by teaching in small steps, perhaps starting with the last step and working back. For example, the child could start with the task of sliding the last piece of a jigsaw into place, with some assistance where necessary. Enormous satisfaction will then be gained by having completed the task and the child will understand the goal of the task being performed as they move to stages further back in the process. These methods can be used at home as well for teaching tasks such as dressing. For example, children can be taught how to put on trousers by teaching the last step first and working back in small stages until the whole task is performed independently.

Staff should be wary of assuming that a child has understood a step in a task that might seem obvious to others. For instance it is useful to check a child's grasp of numbers before moving on to addition and number calculation.

Bearing in mind that many children with Down's syndrome will have short stature and some degree of motor difficulties, consideration should be given to whether the height of activities is practical or whether the child may need a block to stand on. Similarly, can the child's feet touch the floor when sitting or should a block be placed under for desk-based activities? It may be necessary to use a slanted desktop or additional pencil grips to help overcome some motor difficulties. Thought should be given to all equipment that is used in the classroom: the use of old, blunt scissors or half-inflated balls may just compound the child's difficulty and further hamper their progress. The same will apply to computer access, and thought should be given to the size and colour of the pointer as well as the speed at which it moves across the screen. The layout of the computer desktop is today as important as the organisation of the child's desk, and a wealth of adaptive devices and specialist educational software is available to schools and home users.

Speech and language

Children with Down's syndrome often have delayed speech and language skills. Much help and encouragement can be given in this area, and the child will certainly benefit from being amongst other more talkative children. Communication begins at birth, and parents soon begin to recognise their child's hungry and tired cry. Making and encouraging eye contact is important and can be developed within the first three months, by which time babies will usually be returning smiles and making other non-verbal communication. Within the framework of a loving parent–child relationship, communication skills can develop subtly but surely. At first these involve changing facial expressions, gesture and a variety of sounds. Words develop over the first years, unclearly at first, but with recognition and encouragement, more expertly as time goes on. The subtle use of signing can help children to develop their communication skills and word recognition before they are speaking clearly. Children should be encouraged to build up sight vocabulary of single words.

Table showing the rate of acquisition of language skills in Down's syndrome

Activity	Children with DS Average age month	Children with DS Range month	Normal children Average age month	Normal children Range month
Reacts to sounds	1	½–1½		0–1
Turns to sound of voice	7	4–8	4	2–6
Say da-da-, ma-ma	11	7–18	8	5–14
Responds to familiar words	13	10–18	8	5–14
Responds to simple verbal instruction	16	12–24	10	6–14
Jabbers expressively	18	12–30	12	9–18
Says first word(s)	18	13–36	14	10–23
Shows needs by gesture	22	14–30	14½	11–19
A few two-word sentences	30	18–60+		
Uses words spontaneously and to communicate	1½–6 years			

Cunningham, 1982.

The next step is putting ideas and therefore words together in short two- and three-word phrases, and these can be reinforced with the written word. Gradually the building blocks of spoken language and reading come together and the use of language begins to blossom. Language learning is affected by the child's skills in listening, processing and remembering, all of which may be slower to develop in the child with Down's syndrome.

Children with Down's syndrome may, however, continue to show difficulty in acquiring the rules of grammar, which further slows development. As they hear sentences that are more complicated, their difficulties with auditory sequential memory put them at a disadvantage, and focusing on sequencing and memory skills may help to ease the difficulty.

Learning in a language-rich environment will benefit the child's language acquisition considerably.

Children may also have difficulty making clear speech sounds because of low muscle tone or the co-ordination of the speech muscles, which, like other muscles in the body, are affected by the motor dyspraxia in Down's syndrome (see Chapter 6). Exercising the muscles associated with speech can be useful.

- Games which make use of speech sounds can be played to good effect, for example 'p, p, p' copies the sound of a small motor boat and 's, s, s' the sound of a snake.
- Blowing and sucking games, such as using a straw for drinking or 'blow football', strengthen the mouth muscles.
- Playing with a toy telephone will develop the use of, and familiarity with, speech.
- Repeating and rehearsal of nursery and playground rhymes will gradually increase fluency and accustom the child to the natural rhythms of spoken language.

The effect that a large tongue may have on speech development has probably been overemphasised in the past. Efforts to teach the child to keep the tongue inside the mouth are usually successful, although great patience is needed. At school a secret sign, direct to the child, can be employed by the staff, while at home it could be turned into a game, or reminders used, such as stroking downwards under a child's chin. All the exercises mentioned in this section will gradually increase the child's mouth and tongue control and improve articulation.

The use of signing will often avoid the frustration caused by communication difficulties, and signing can be introduced very early, often in the first year or two. When it is combined with spoken language, the development of communication and language skills is encouraged. The child who learns to love books is often the child who is likely to have the least trouble recognising pictures and, later, words. Teachers will be encouraged to learn that teaching children to read also improves their language concepts and therefore speech. The words they learn to read are the words most likely to emerge in spoken language. Occasionally, children with Down's syndrome will have greater difficulty with reading, and this

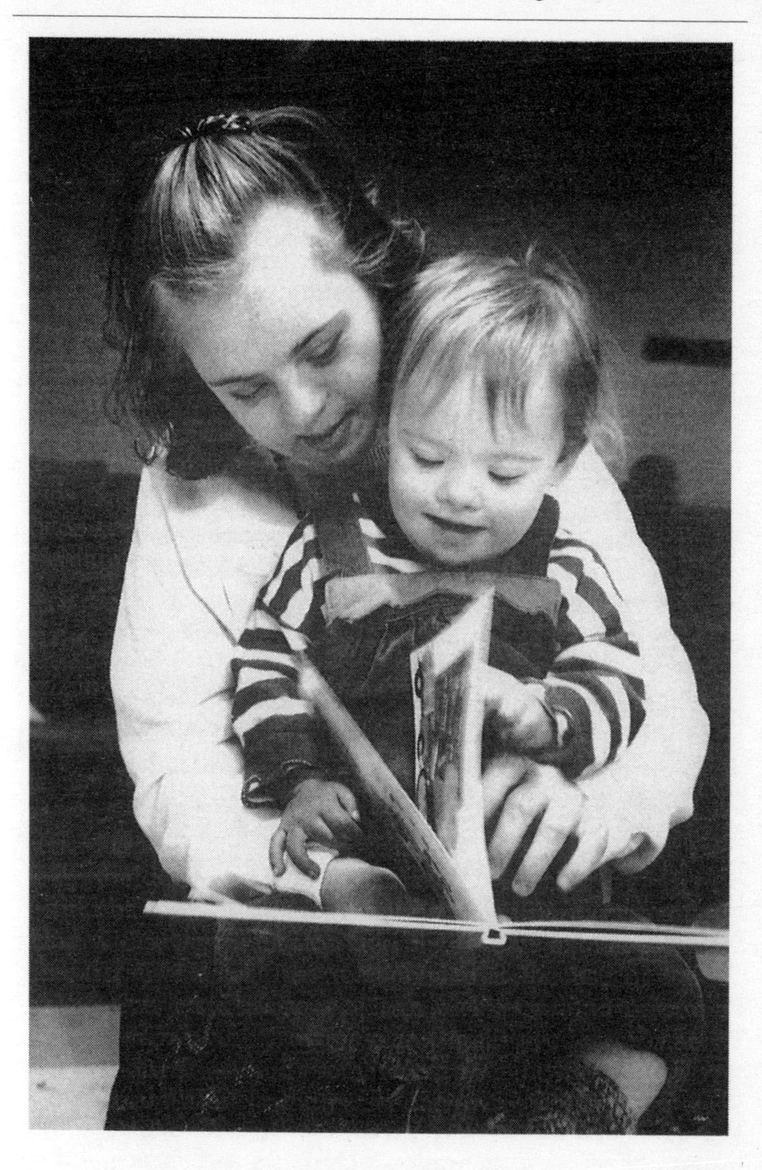

Most children with Down's syndrome will be able to read and write when they are older. They should be encouraged to explore books from an early age.

needs to be discussed with the teacher and support staff. As with all children final success in reading will vary greatly.

The intelligibility of the speech of adolescents with Down's syndrome

	Girls		Boys	
	Under 14	Over 14	Under 14	Over 14
Parents usually understand	88%	86%	86%	73%
Strangers usually understand	45%	32%	10%	18%

From Buckley & Sacks, 1986

It should be borne in mind that extra patience on the part of listeners may be required when the child is trying to speak. Expressive language is of vital importance to any child and nothing is more frustrating than not being able to put ideas and points of view to other people. Great patience is required to ensure that a language-impaired child is not discouraged from attempting to speak. Staff should always listen carefully and ensure that the child is given plenty of opportunity to attempt to answer questions and join in discussions, allowing extra time to get a response and contribution from the child.

It takes a while for children with Down's syndrome to find the confidence to put their ideas into words, so it helps if the rest of the group or class are encouraged to be patient. After a while teachers get much better insight into a child's attempts at speaking and very soon become as good as the child's parents at understanding what is being said.

Currently, a high proportion of adults with Down's syndrome have difficulty in making themselves understood to strangers, and about 30 per cent have stammering or stuttering as a symptom. Relaxation techniques and speech and lan guage therapy advice may be of help in these cases.

With the advent of modern technology, far more teaching opportunities and communication aids are becoming available to people with continuing communication difficulties. This technology, however, cannot really match the value of a language-rich environment and the loving encouragement of parents, carers and interested teachers.

Dexterity

Difficulties with dexterity and coordination can present problems when children with Down's syndrome first go to school or playschool, and it can be some time before a child can give attention to two separate activities at the same time, for example walking and putting on gloves at the same time, or talking and eating. However, this is often what is expected at school, for example using one hand to steady some bricks while using another hand to add bricks to the pile. Some approaches that may be useful in encouraging dexterity are as follows:

- A reminder of which hand to use – children with Down's syndrome can get confused about which is their dominant hand.
- Fine motor difficulties may make it hard to learn to hold a pen or pencil. Finger grip can be improved by playing games that require the child to pick up progressively smaller objects from a container, using finger and thumb. Squeezy balls, pick-up objects and games can be stored in a box and the 'finger gym' activities varied at different times of day.
- Finger-game rhymes will also help to strengthen the fingers and encourage them to move individually. Fine control of the fingers is not possible for a child who is seated and whose feet are dangling. Provision of a footrest is essential for such activities.
- Scissors are best controlled if they are held with the forefinger along the shaft and the second or third finger in the lower finger hole. Trainer scissors, with two sets of finger holes, are often easier for the child to manipulate.
- If buttons are difficult, re-sewing them with a longer shank can ease the problem.
- Exercises, ball games and computer skills can be used to increase and improve hand–eye coordination.

Children with Down's syndrome will need plenty of encouragement with fine motor skills and particularly with writing.

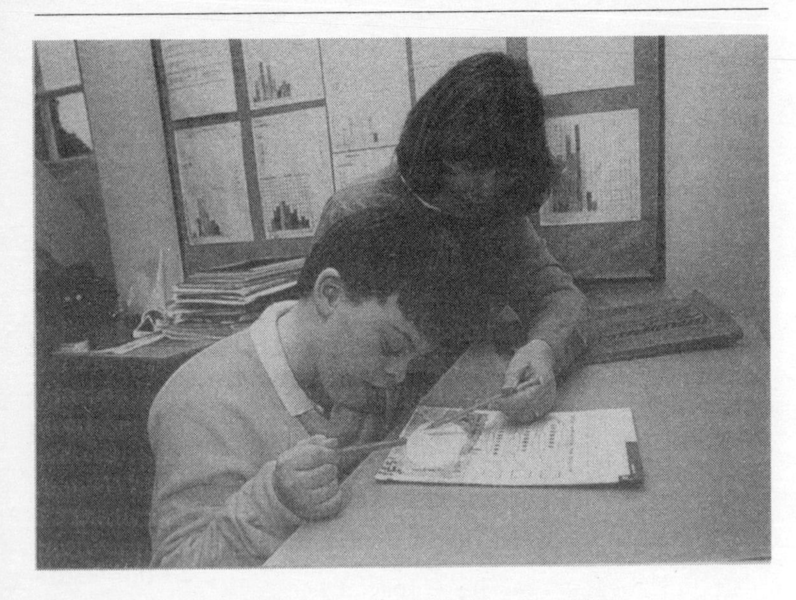

Drawing and cutting out – to encourage fine motor skills.

Despite the fact that pencil control may be difficult, if writing is taught carefully from the start, much can be achieved.

Concentration

Children with Down's syndrome can have difficulty concentrating on the same task for long periods, and it can be sensible to limit activities to shorter periods than is the norm in order to avoid frustration. The child can then be encouraged to spend a little longer at activities with a simple reward system (rewards can range from a smile or a word of praise to a treat), and gradually the child's concentration span will increase; all concerned should maintain a reasonable but high expectation and work towards achievable goals in this area.

Recreation and break-times

Much has been said about the importance of free play at break-times and lunchtimes for school children, when children have a chance to get away from the structure and discipline of the classroom. Play times offer a chance for genuine peer-to-peer interaction, and the role of the support assistant should be limited to ensuring that the child is able to take part positively and perhaps to set up and structure games that involve other children that are physically within the scope of the child with Down's syndrome. Not all children want to join in everything all of the time: observation and time out are useful activities in themselves.

Today's child

Today school children with Down's syndrome have a very different lot from that of their counterparts 10 or 15 years ago. They are generally very much a part of the family and society in which they live. They join in and are included in all areas of family and school life. Typically, children are entering community playgroups and nurseries, attending their local mainstream school and joining in social activities with siblings and friends who do not have special needs.

Increasingly, children and adults with Down's syndrome are being recognised as people in their own right, able to participate in meaningful ways in the life of their communities. Each year more young adults with Down's syndrome are living in the community, gaining qualifications and experiences, and succeeding in a wide variety of ordinary jobs.

Connexions

This is the government's support service for all young people aged 13 to 19 in England. The service aims to provide integrated advice, guidance and access to personal development opportunities for this group and to help them make a smooth transition to adulthood and working life. The success of Connexions depends on the involvement of young people – listening to and taking account of their views. Connexions joins up the work of six government Departments and their agencies and organisations on the ground, together with private and voluntary sector groups and youth and careers services. It brings together all the services and support young people need during their teenage years. It offers practical help with choosing the right courses and careers, including access to broader personal development through activities such as sport, performing arts and volunteering activities. It will also provide help and advice on issues such as drug abuse, sexual health and homelessness.

Connexions is being delivered through local Partnerships working to national planning guidance. The Partnerships will cover the same geographical areas as the Learning and Skills Councils. They will have flexibility to meet local needs using the design that works best. All young people will have access to a personal adviser. For some young people this may be just for careers advice, for others it may involve more in-depth support to help identify barriers to learning and find solutions, brokering access to more specialist support. This applies particularly to young people with Down's syndrome. The personal advisers will work in a range of settings: schools, colleges, one-stop shops, community centres and on an outreach basis. As teenagers near the end of their secondary school placement Connexions will help pave part of the way into adult life.

9

Growing up and adult life

This chapter will look at the growing opportunities for people with Down's syndrome as they reach adulthood. Medical, social and legal aspects will all be examined.

Life expectancy

It is now clear that the life expectancy of people with Down's syndrome is greater than previously believed. Institutional life no doubt led to less than optimal care in some cases, and exaggerated the risk of infectious diseases being passed from one to another. Now that people with Down's syndrome are brought up and live in the community, there is a far more optimistic outlook.

The major determinant of mortality in the first three decades, and particularly in the first year, of life is the presence of congenital heart disease. Over 90 per cent of children without a heart problem survive the first year, whereas about 25 per cent of those with congenital heart disease will die in infancy. A study from British Columbia reviewed the life expectancy of 1,341 people with Down's syndrome; for those with congenital heart disease survival to age five was 62 per cent, to age 10 was 57 per cent, to age 20 was 53 per cent, and to age 30 was 50 per cent. For those without congenital heart anomalies the corresponding figures showed survival to age five in 87 per cent, to age 10 in 85 per cent, to age 20 in 82 per cent and to 30 in 79 per cent.

Disordered immunity still accounts for a number of early deaths, and after the age of 40 the emergence of Alzheimer's disease tends to give a life expectancy less than that expected with other mentally disabling conditions. A study based at Stoke Park Hospital, in Bristol, between 1976 and 1980 showed that the average life expectancy of people with

Down's syndrome was 55 for men and 53 for women. A recent Australian study showed an improvement to 58 years of age. Clearly, when plans are being drawn up for financial provision, social support and housing of people with Down's syndrome, statistics like this need bearing in mind.

Biological maturation

Information on the physical and sexual maturation of adolescents with Down's syndrome is limited, and until recently has largely related to those living in institutional care, where reported abnormalities seemed common. More recent studies have been on home-reared children, with fewer abnormalities being seen.

Biological maturation in males with Down's syndrome

The development of secondary sexual characteristics (those that appear at puberty) in males with Down's syndrome is essentially the same as that in the general population. There is normal development of pubic hair, but beard growth is on the whole slower than in the general population. There is a tendency for testicular size to be smaller, but many men with Down's syndrome have normally sized testicles. Similarly, stretched penile length tends to be shorter.

Early studies may have overestimated the prevalence of genital abnormalities in boys. The previously quoted incidence of undescended testicles has been as high as 50 per cent. One recent study of home-reared children with Down's syndrome from Maryland showed two of 53 to have perineal hypospadias (where the urinary opening is not at the end of the penis but at its base), two with bilaterally undescended testicles and five with retractile testicles. These findings are probably more representative of the actual prevalence.

Study of endocrine function has also shown conflicting results. Plasma testosterone (the sex hormone leading to masculine features) has on the whole been shown to be normal, but a number of studies have shown a significant number of boys to have raised levels of follicle stimulating hormone and luteinising hormone. These two hormones are produced by the pituitary gland, follicle stimulating hormone stimulating sperm production. These results are found before and after puberty, and suggest a partial primary gonadal dysfunction. Studies suggest that this may progress with age, and degenerative change has been seen in some testes examined histologically. There may be inefficient feedback between the gonads and the hypothalamic–pituitary axis (the way the gonad and brain interact to secure normal hormone levels) or a lack of target organ response to circulating stimulating hormone (page 64). The disordered membrane function referred to Chapter 2 on biochemical genetics, is probably also important in this respect.

Data on spermatogenesis (sperm production by the testes) are limited because of the problems of sperm collection for laboratory study. It does appear that there is reduced fertility in a high proportion of males with Down's syndrome. Where sperm counts are normal, motility is often poor and the proportion of abnormal forms high. Nevertheless, males with Down's syndrome cannot be assumed to be sterile; 1990 saw the first report of a pregnancy where the father was confirmed to be a man with Down's syndrome.

Biological maturation in females with Down's syndrome

The development of secondary sexual characteristics in females is the same as in the general population, although there are reports of axillary (armpit) hair in females being lost at a relatively early age and a relative lack of apocrine (sweat) glands in the axilla.

Although the onset of menstruation is a little delayed in Down's syndrome, it is by no more than a few months, and the differences are unimportant. In other respects the characteristics of the menstrual cycle are the same as for all women.

Whether ovulation occurs is more difficult to establish. Studies seem to show that about a third of women with Down's syndrome show a definite pattern of ovulation, a third no evidence of ovulation and in about a third the evidence is indeterminate.

The number of reported cases of pregnancy in women with Down's syndrome is strikingly low. To date there have been

30 reported pregnancies occurring in 26 women. Hormonal studies show the same elevated serum levels of FSH and LH as in men, implying a similar primary gonadal dysfunction.

Self-esteem

Adolescence should not only be a time for physical development but also one for emotional maturation. Disabled children are more vulnerable to a variety of psycho-social problems, and parents and carers need to be aware of this so that they may encourage confidence and independence rather than reinforcing a sense of separateness and the need constantly to rely on others.

From quite an early age children with Down's syndrome will be aware that they are different in many ways from other children. This sense of being different in some way may be seen for the first time when children enter nursery school and feel the pressure of children the same age as themselves communicating freely and generally performing more adeptly. After a while they may become aware or perceive that their peers have negative feelings towards them. The fact that others react in this way may lead to feelings of hurt. Through this exposure to other people outside the immediate family, children with Down's syndrome gradually perceive that others consider them to be different and inferior. Security comes from a feeling of belonging and being similar to others; when these feelings are absent the effect can be upsetting.

Within society there is a considerable tolerance of disability, but beneath the surface there is often an involuntary rejection. (It is this feeling of rejection that first confronts parents following the birth of their child with Down's syndrome.) The expression of these mixed emotions can be confusing. At times children with Down's syndrome may be subjected to overt kindness; at other times to frank embarrassment.

Negative attitudes towards disabled people have been shown to increase with age in children. When they are very young they do not mind playing with disabled children, but as they grow older they slowly show a greater intolerance. This is because of the essential part of growing up already referred to: that of a feeling of similarity with one's peers; to be seen to befriend a disabled child may be seen as socially disadvantageous in a peer group. Gradually as they get older children with Down's syndrome realise they are being avoided because of their disability. Or to put that another way, all people, including children, tend to make friends with people of similar ability and unwittingly leave out people of lesser ability. This gradual growth in awareness of society's norms unfortunately often leads to feelings of self-rejection. The inability to change the impairment leads to feelings of inferiority, and causes the self-image to alter and self-esteem to fall. With increasing maturity young people with Down's syndrome can even start to assume that they are disabled because they have done something wrong, which in turn can lead to feelings of guilt.

Nonetheless, it must be noted that the ever-increasing numbers of children with Down's syndrome attending mainstream schools have led to a new generation of people growing up alongside people with Down's syndrome who do not see a problem. This has also been reflected in people with Down's syndrome living and working in the community. They are visible and known and liked by the people around them. This is one of the very positive effects of inclusive policies. Segregation enforces negative stereotypes, fear and hostility. Segregation is now disappearing from our society.

Parents have a central role in promoting independence and confidence in their children. Overprotectiveness can lead to infantilisation (persistently treating a child like a baby) and to problems with self-help, self-reliance and inadequacy. Worse, if parents show themselves to be embarrassed or to reject their children in company, the child with Down's syndrome will have additional problems with self-esteem, feeling that they have failed their parents. These thoughts can lead in turn to social isolation and depression, with an ultimate detrimental effect on performance.

Research has also shown that people with Down's syndrome who have their condition explained to them have higher levels of self-esteem than those who have had no explanation but perhaps have heard these two words throughout their lives. Many families find it helpful to explain Down's syndrome to their children from quite an early age. On school entry they are often content to hear that they find it more difficult to learn some things than many other children and that is why they need some extra help. If that message is repeated over the years – but always balanced by praise for achievement and opportunities to do things they find easier – then it becomes an accepted fact of life. As the years go by, the term Down's syndrome can be introduced, pointing out that there are many other young people with the same condition. The DSA's *Down 2 Earth* magazine, written by people with Down's syndrome for people with Down's syndrome, can be a helpful source of information and promotes a feeling of belonging.

Parents need to show warmth and sympathetic support, tempered by firmness, when their child shrinks from a task they are probably capable of. Talking to their child about difficulties should reduce tension. The children themselves, where possible, should be encouraged to talk to others about this too. This can reduce discomfort, anxiety and uncertainty when new friendships are being made and new situations entered. Ability should be emphasised rather than disability, and a balance should be struck in life whereby enjoyable tasks are pursued in order to balance those things a child finds difficult.

Doctors can be guilty of showing disproportionate attention to purely medical aspects of a child's condition, whilst ignoring the psycho-social consequences. It is these aspects of a child's life that may prove to be the most disadvantageous, and to maintain good standards of medical care they need to be addressed.

Friendships

Adolescence is usually a time for moving away from the family, increasing independence and creating friendships. However, although teenagers with Down's syndrome have the usual range of teenage interests – pop stars, music and sport – they rarely seem able to pursue these interests outside the home with friends of their own age. Instead they tend to spend their time watching the TV or listening to tapes or records. Most are very dependent on their families for social activity.

Much of this social isolation arises out of poor communication skills. Although the speech in four out of five teenagers with Down's syndrome is easily understood by their family, only 30 per cent of girls and 14 per cent of boys are easily understood by strangers. In one survey, only one in three had a good friend, and half the girls and a third of the boys saw their friends less than once a week. This loneliness can lead to the creation of imaginary friends in roughly half of teenagers with Down's syndrome, this pattern of behaviour often being established at quite an early age. Conversations may be held with these fantasy friends. This, along with imaginative play with dolls and similar toys, seems to help teenagers work out things that are bothering them. It must be understood that although this behaviour is not age appropriate, it does not represent a psychosis – psychotic behaviour is actually very rare in Down's syndrome.

Research in the United States has shown that self-talk is actually healthy in the vast majority of cases. It is often the way people with Down's syndrome think things through, where other people will internalise these thoughts. Adults can use this play as a cue to help young people with Down's syndrome to overcome some of their worries.

Much can be done to help loneliness and encourage integration by imaginative enterprise on the part of parents to find social outlets outside the home, and by continuing efforts to improve communication skills. For example in Britain, Mencap run Gateway clubs, which allow even the more severely disabled an opportunity to socialise with others, some of whom will be more and some less disabled than them. A number of charitable organisations and some local authorities run Outreach clubs, where the emphasis is on social integration, with trips to local restaurants or places of interest. Cubs, Brownies, Scouts and Guides all offer places to young people with Down's syndrome, as do many keep-fit and martial arts centres. The Uphill Ski Club was founded with the disabled in mind, and many Outward Bound centres run courses for the disabled too. Many people with Down's syndrome are participating in inclusive activities with their peers. It has been found on many occasions that strong friendships have been formed through sharing common interests and hobbies.

Success in many of these ventures depends on a 'buddy' system, whereby a more able person will befriend, encourage and support a disabled person. The Ocean Youth Club is a good example of this, where a number of learning-disabled people have had an introduction to sailing. In the USA a number of neighbourhood 'buddy' schemes have grown up where this sort of encouragement and support is pursued on a community basis. Both those with and those without learning disability voice the benefits they have derived from the schemes, which often lead to feelings of mutual respect and lasting friendships.

Love and marriage

People with Down's syndrome are sexual beings and have the same needs and desires as the rest of the population. What is imperative is that people with Down's syndrome receive good sex education.

Families may need advice on how to control behaviour perceived by others to be sexual. Children should be taught that masturbation is something to be done in private and that, after a certain age, hugging and kissing as a show of affection is not socially acceptable where strangers are involved.

Some adults with Down's syndrome will, of course, mature to a degree whereby they develop a friendship with another person and go on to have a sexual relationship. A small number of people with Down's syndrome marry, and this number is likely to increase. This sort of development will need a lot of support from family, friends and society. In a changing world it is likely to be seen with ever-increasing frequency as appropriate support reaches more people with Down's syndrome, allowing them to reach their true potential.

Down's syndrome and the law

As people with Down's syndrome achieve better lifestyles for themselves, they will be increasingly expected to make choices, take risks and be responsible for the consequences of personal decisions. Even quite severely impaired people may be able to make simple choices where the issues are explained carefully in appropriate language. The mental impairment, of course, makes them more vulnerable to exploitation by the unscrupulous; they can often be persuaded where biased information is given.

The issue of consent

First of all a piece of history, as we look back at how the law has changed in the past 50 years to reflect changes in society.

Section 7 of the Sexual Offences Act 1956 states that it is an offence for a man to have unlawful sexual intercourse with a woman who is a 'mental defective', where 'unlawful' means 'outside marriage', and 'defective' means 'a person suffering from a state of arrested or incomplete development of mind that includes severe impairment of intelligence and social functioning'. It seems unlikely that a woman with Down's syndrome who has severe learning difficulties could ever validly consent to marriage, even if the opportunity arose, so lawful sex in this context seems only possible where the man was himself incapable of realising her state of impairment. As the purpose of this Act is to protect vulnerable women who might be exploited, prosecution would no doubt be pursued only very selectively.

Parents of the more severely learning-disabled young women with Down's syndrome are often rightly worried about their daughters' vulnerability to pregnancy, and a number of sterilisations have been carried out for this reason (at least 36 girls under 18 were sterilised in England in 1973 to 1974, and in 1987 the Department of Health stated that around 90 sterilisations were performed each year on women aged under 19). Previously, before proceeding with the sterilisation, medical practitioners would share the particular issues of individual cases with the girl herself (if possible), and the girl's parents, social workers and other health care professionals. Under the Mental Health Act 1959, consent could be given on behalf of the individual concerned. This followed the notion that guardianship could be held not only by parents but also by personnel of social services.

The Mental Health Act 1983 replaced this 1959 Act, and significantly restricted the role of guardians in this respect. In particular, they could no longer sign consent forms and this, together with the case of Re B (a minor) heard before the Court of Appeal in 1987, has given learning-disabled people a new status in law. Now those with learning difficulties who have enough understanding to give consent to a particular procedure are allowed to do so (previously this was not possible; the guardian had to be asked). Proxy consent is no longer valid in law (see below). This is a welcome development in view of the increasing amount of community care, the rejection of the concept of infantilism and a greater social awareness of human rights on the part of people with learning difficulties.

The problem then remained of how to organise the medical care of those who were unable to understand the issues involved. When treatment was not controversial, doctors were authorised to go ahead, if possible with the agreement (but not the consent) of the parents or usual caretakers of the child. In these circumstances doctors were acting 'in good faith' and showing a 'duty of care'. In an emergency doctors might clearly intervene without the consent of the person involved or the support of close relatives, as the 'principle of necessity' is recognised in law.

The situation got complicated where the medical procedure involved was of a controversial nature, such as sterilisation. In Re B (a minor) the Court of Appeal authorised an operation to sterilise a learning-disabled girl of 17. The girl, known as Jeanette, was said to have a mental age of five or six and to be incapable of understanding the procedure of sterilisation, and therefore not able to give informed consent herself. Lord Justice Dillon said that the Court had jurisdiction to authorise a sterilisation operation on a ward of court (which Jeanette was) in wardship proceedings, but it was a jurisdiction that should be exercised only as a last resort when all other forms of contraception had been considered. It was added that there was no question of a natural parent or local authority with parental rights giving consent to a sterilisation operation without first obtaining the leave of the Court.

In reaching its decision the Court had considered an earlier much publicised case, that of Re D (a minor) 1976. This related to an 11-year-old girl with Sotos syndrome who was said to have an IQ of 80 and had a behaviour disorder. Her widowed mother feared that she might become pregnant. Local doctors agreed, but an educational psychologist challenged the appropriateness of this decision. Mrs Justice Heilbron heard that the proposed operation involved the deprivation of a woman's basic human rights to reproduce. Furthermore, if the operation were performed on a woman for non-therapeutic reasons and without her consent, it would be a violation of that right. It was further ruled that such decisions should not be within the doctor's sole clinical judgement and that in the evidence the operation was neither medically indicated nor necessary and would not be in the girl's best interest. Each case would have to be decided by a court on its merits and on the evidence.

In 1989 five law lords found that the 'principle of necessity' should be stretched to controversial situations such as sterilisation. The interpretation is that doctors should act in accordance with a substantial body of medical opinion or be seen to be following the established medical practice of the day so that they might be 'acting in the best interest of the patient'. It is clear from this judgement that when a medical intervention is planned that might be deemed controversial, doctors would be prudent to gain the agreement from a court so that the anticipated controversial intervention 'will not be unlawful'.

This position was clarified in 1995 when the Law Commission produced guidance in the form of a Code of Practice on mental capacity and consent. They noted that decisions should be made with people, not for them. Good practice therefore involves investment in time and communication with the person concerned and carers. Information should be given in broad terms, in simple language and using visual aids and signing as necessary. It should not be assumed that capacity or lack of capacity in respect to one area equates directly to another situation. For example, the ability to consent to medical treatment may not mean that an adult is able to give their consent to sexual activity. This approach to the assessment of capacity can be regarded as a 'functional approach'.

When a competent person refuses consent this should be respected unless circumstances warrant the use of the Mental Health Act 1983, which is only applicable to the assessment and treatment of mental disorder. In law no one, not even parents or medical staff, can consent on behalf of an adult who is not competent to give consent. It is the responsibility of the treatment provider to determine the person's competence to give consent, and The Mental Health Act Code of Practice (Department of Health and Welsh Office 1993) describes the questions to be asked to determine competency.

The Health Service Guidelines on consent, HSG(90)22, are accompanied by a handbook, 'A guide to consent for examination and treatment', and the model consent forms were revised in HSG(92)32. The General Medical Council, British Medical Association and Royal College of Nursing also produce guidance. Specialist learning disability professionals should be able to advise the staff of general NHS services.

Usually, if the person is not competent to give consent, treatment is lawful provided it is in the person's best interests. The criteria for determining this are also in The Mental Health Act Code of Practice. In many cases it is not only lawful to treat an individual unable to give consent but it is common law duty to do so. However, certain forms of treatment that give rise to special concern, such as sterilisation, should be referred to Court.

This approach focuses on the decision itself and the capability of the person concerned to understand, at the time it is made, the nature of the decision required and its implications. This approach is very specific and avoids generalisations that may involve unnecessary intrusions into the affairs of the person. Workers will need to determine whether the vulnerable adult is making the decision of their own free will or whether they are being subjected to coercion or intimidation. If the latter is suspected, efforts should be made to offer the adult 'distance' from the situation to help decision-making.

Three other important pieces of legislation are relevant in this context:

European Convention on the Protection of Human Rights 1950

This Convention gives the individual basic rights and freedoms under European law. The individual's rights have to be respected by others, including government agencies. It is a statement of values and standards that have to be kept by European governments. It covers many rights and freedoms, including the right to life, a fair trial, privacy, and freedom of expression and thought. The European Court of Human Rights in Strasbourg hears human rights cases.

UN Convention on the Rights of the Child 1989

This Convention ensures that the rights of children, including disabled children, are recognised in international law. It includes the right of disabled children to special care, education and training to enable them to lead a full and active life.

Children have a right to:

- express their views;
- be allowed freedom of expression, thought and association;
- be free from discrimination, inhumane treatment, all forms of violence and unlawful restrictions on liberty;
- information, education and health care.

Human Rights Act 1998

The Human Rights Act 1998 came into effect in October 2000. It brings into UK law the European Convention on Human Rights. This means that anyone wishing to make a claim under the European Convention will avoid the cost and delay of taking a case to the European Court in Strasburg.

The Act means that public authorities such as health providers and local authorities must act in a manner that is compatible with Convention rights. This includes NHS doctors and other health workers, social services and social work departments.

At the time of writing the Mental Capacity Bill (currently termed Incapacity Bill) is the subject of revision at Committee stage. It is to be hoped that this development will offer the learning-disabled more power and freedom than ever before to determine their own destiny.

The law and hospitalisation

The Mental Health Act 1983 was an update of previously existing legislation, but unfortunately still confuses the issue of mental illness and learning disability. Where compulsory admission to hospital is concerned, the law talks of a central concept of 'mental impairment' (arrested or incomplete development of the mind). Very few people with Down's syndrome are abnormally aggressive or seriously irresponsible, and it is only these who could be compulsorily admitted or detained in hospital because of 'mental disorder', and then it would be for a non-renewable period (maximum 28 days).

Following detention, hospitalisation is for the person's health or safety or for the protection of other people. The admission is for treatment which is designed 'to alleviate or prevent any serious deterioration of the patient's condition'. The patient must be mentally impaired such that hospital care and treatment are appropriate, and it must be impossible to provide this care and treatment elsewhere. A person's nearest relative or an approved social worker can apply for the person's admission, which is based upon two medical recommendations. If the hospital accepts, the patient is detained for up to six months, a period that is then renewable.

In England and Wales doctors can renew a detention order initially for six months and thereafter annually, although this is only if the conditions that were pertinent to the initial admission still apply. However, where the person involved has severe learning difficulties, it must be established that care could not be provided in a different community setting. People can apply to the Mental Health Review Tribunal, which can order the patient to be discharged if the conditions are not fulfilled. When the person involved is not capable of appealing themselves, there is a statutory requirement of hospital managers to apply to the Tribunal on their behalf at three-yearly intervals. With the advent of community care, providing it is adequately resourced, long-term detention of this sort should disappear; hospitalisation should then only be required where danger is involved.

In practice very few people in England are admitted or detained under the provisions of this Act. Where compulsory admission is undertaken, it is usually by use of short-term powers, where the protections for the 'patients' are fewer. The first of these is a 28-day order, where the patient must be suffering from a mental disorder (see above). The conditions for admission are not as stringent as those already considered, but the patient does have a right of appeal within 14 days. A 72-hour order can be used for admission for assessment in an emergency; the same conditions apply, but the agreement of only one doctor is required. Down's syndrome itself does not predispose to conditions that lead to admission of this sort, except under very rare circumstances; this is where mental illness exists alongside the learning disability, and treatment is required as it would be in the general population.

Thankfully most admissions and detentions are through informal admission procedures on a voluntary basis. The problem is that, where learning disability is concerned, the people concerned are vulnerable to suggestion that is not necessarily in their own interest; the naïvety of people with learning difficulties can be misused in a deceitful way. In the past there have been many instances of misleading, unfair or even unkind treatment in institutional care. These situations are now rare with care in the community. Furthermore, the new regulations reduce the powers of guardianship and this should reduce the burden on local authorities, since the regulations no longer imply a parental role. People with Down's syndrome should now be able to live in a reasonable fashion in the community without too many restrictions upon their freedom and with institutionalisation avoided. Further aspects of the law and people with Down's syndrome are considered in the sections on education and in Chapter 10, where the rights to life and to treatment are also considered.

The Children Act 1989 is the most comprehensive piece of legislation enacted about children and replaces the previously fragmented pieces of legislation as a comprehensive statement of the law relating to the care and protection of children. One of the most important principles behind the Act is that the welfare of the child is paramount and that children are generally best looked after within their own family. Where other agencies are required to supervise the care of the child, it is stated that this is best done in the context of a partnership between those agencies and the family concerned. Much of the Act deals with the issue of child protection, but important consideration is also given to children with disabilities. It is hoped that the creation of the joint register of disabled children between health, education and social services will greatly facilitate the identification, registration and a co-ordinated provision of services. This applies not only at any early stage when assessments were being drawn up and procedures defined in the 1996 Education Act (see above) but also in relation to the provision of respite care and the subsequent placement of adults with severe learning difficulties in residential community houses.

Integration, education and employment prospects

With the closure of the large long-stay residential hospitals ten years or so ago, the rule is that adults with Down's syndrome will find themselves supported in community houses, either living alone or with a small number of people of similar ability. Even for those adults with Down's syndrome who are less able, very sheltered environments or special-care facilities are available so that care is provided in the comfort of a small unit with a homely environment.

For the more able, greater integration into the community will require further education, particularly in relation to developing independence skills. Currently only about one in six young adults with Down's syndrome go to further education colleges on life-skill courses, but it is likely that this proportion will increase. Given adequate interest on the part of the staff, and adequate resources, much can be achieved, even with the more severely learning-disabled.

A good example of this is a study carried out at the Universities of Minnesota and Maryland. The study described how a 16-year-old youth with severe learning difficulties was taught over a six-week period how to use a local bowling alley. Such language as he had was unintelligible, but he was shown how to overcome this problem by the use of cards expressing simple wishes. It was not long before he learnt who he needed to see for appropriate footwear and the bowls, and, after an enjoyable game, how to use the food and drink vending machines. The skills acquired in this setting were clearly useful to the young man in other circumstances too. This shows how, if people are imaginative and are not confined by prejudgements, much can be achieved for those with learning difficulties in society.

Currently, about 75 per cent of adults with Down's syndrome go to Day Centres or sheltered workshops. There are advantages to this arrangement; it structures the day for the people involved, and they have an opportunity to develop friendships with people of similar ability. However, the tasks available to them are often rather mundane, and the environment is often not rich enough for many to reach their natural full potential.

It is disappointing to learn that only about 1 per cent of adults with Down's syndrome are in gainful employment. This is far fewer than would be expected if one predicts the potential usefulness of people of their ability. A wide range of unskilled and semi-skilled jobs are within the intellectual competence of most school-leavers with Down's syndrome –

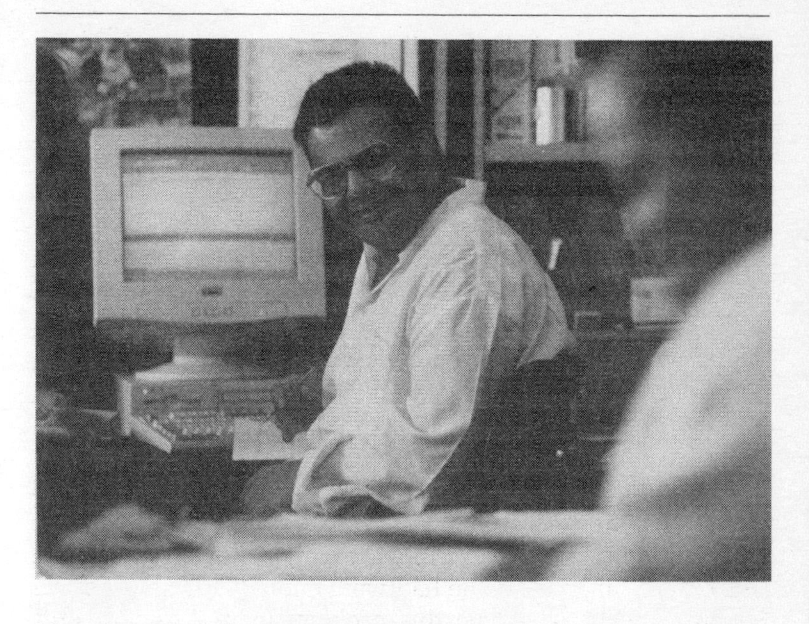

More than ever before young people with Down's syndrome have the opportunity for further education ...

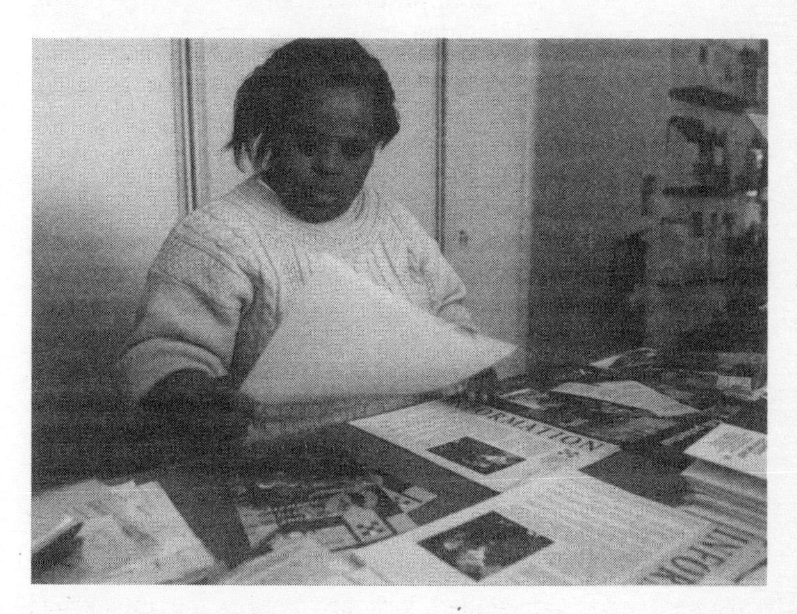

... and employment.

kitchen work, gardening, portering and positions in retail are but a few examples. As employees, people with Down's syndrome often prove to be more punctual, reliable and malleable than other people employed in the same type of work.

Disability Rights Commission

The Disability Rights Commission has now been set up and is working towards ending discrimination against disabled people. It promotes equal opportunities for disabled people, encourages good practice in the treatment of disabled people and reviews the working of the Disability Discrimination Act (DDA).

The DDA is designed to stop people and businesses from discriminating against disabled people. It covers:

- Employment – employers are not allowed to discriminate against disabled people and have to make 'reasonable adjustments' to the workplace. However, this does not apply to organisations with fewer than 15 employees.
- Goods, services and facilities – refusing to serve disabled customers is illegal unless 'justified'. Since October 1999 policies and practices have had to be changed if they discriminate against disabled people, and aids should be provided where 'reasonable'. From 2004 changes to premises will also have to be considered.
- Renting or buying properties – landlords, estate agents and management committees of domestic properties must not discriminate against disabled people without justification. There is no requirement on them to make changes to premises.
- Education – since September 2002 schools, colleges and universities have not been allowed to discriminate against prospective or existing disabled pupils or students.
- Transport – the Government has powers to set minimum access rules for new public transport vehicles, including buses, taxis and trains.
- Cases that go to court will help decide what changes or practices are 'reasonable' or when discriminatory treatment is 'justified'.

The acquisition of employment does much to enhance the life

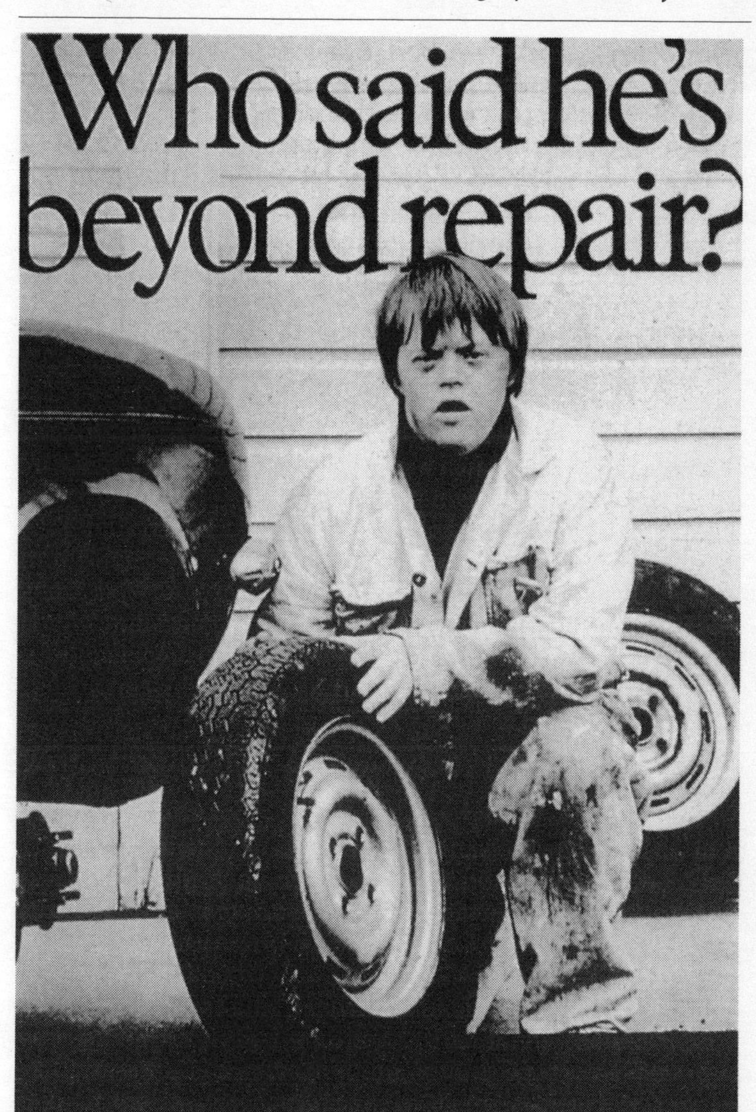
Who said he's
beyond repair?

of any adult. Apart from structuring the day and improving self-esteem, it enhances income, which in turn brings the opportunity to improve other aspects of life, particularly the opportunity to live alone, or at least with a smaller number of people rather than living communally in a community house. For those from richer families this ideal may be secured through private means, but for most much reliance will be placed on local authority facilities. Facilities are very variable from one region to another. The best model for care seems to be for local self-help groups for the disabled to liaise with local and education authorities so that duplication of effort is avoided. In so doing, young adults with Down's syndrome must be encouraged to speak for themselves and to achieve a degree of self-determination. Key workers are allocated to individual families and the quagmire of undue bureaucracy is simplified. It is likely that in the future we shall see the inadequate resources allocated by central government funds bolstered by funds raised in the charitable and private sector. The final result should be better facilities for our adult learning-disabled population.

In summary, it can be said that the last few decades have brought greater acknowledgment of the need for self-determination of people with learning disabilities. The next few decades will see the fulfilment of that ideal, with a greater number living independently in the community, with access to work appropriate to their level of ability, which in turn will secure an enhancement of the quality of their lives.

Changes of this sort require extra resources and careful preparation. Sadly, many local authorities have been under-resourced in this respect. Now that a much better pattern of community care has been defined, it is to be hoped the political will is retained to achieve it.

10

Hopes and fears

Birth and the right to life

A number of children with Down's syndrome are born with life-threatening conditions, some remediable and some irremediable. Where the problem cannot be helped, adequate support for the family and good nursing care is what is required.

When a baby with Down's syndrome is born with a remediable medical problem, such as certain heart conditions or duodenal atresia, a potential area of conflict between parents and health care professionals arises. The medical and nursing staff have a duty to remedy the problem and preserve life. The parents may see this as their 'way out', confronted as they are by their initial sense of uncertainty and a fear of what the future holds for them. The thought that the problem might be allowed to go away holds some attraction. They are already in the throes of grieving for the child who did not arrive, and the thought that nature might actually relieve them of the problem before it has become burdensome can be quite comforting.

At times in the past doctors have held much sympathy with the feelings of parents in this situation, to the point where they have allowed children to die, or even secured a child's death by means of sedation. The doctors have considered undesirable the thought of parents having to cope with the handicap, and have also held a view that they are perhaps saving the children themselves some unhappiness, if not suffering, by securing their demise. The sedated babies failed to demand feeds and died within a few days of birth.

In the 1980's a consultant paediatrician was charged with murder (R. v. Arthur) in circumstances similar to these. In the course of the trial, the charge was replaced by one of attempted murder as more forensic evidence was submitted, and ultimately the defendant was found not guilty. Although the trial left many important legal and ethical principles unaddressed, it did make it clear that juries are quite disinclined to find doctors guilty of murder in these circumstances. More recently still (Re C, a minor), a judge found that it would be 'not unlawful' to let a child die where severe disability existed and where suffering would be avoided.

Whereas there are many situations in medicine where it can readily be seen that to prolong life would be wrong in terms of common ethics and humanity, the diagnosis of Down's syndrome alone at birth could never justify this. At this stage future development cannot be predicted. Most parents would be able to hope for a child who at worst would have a moderate learning disability. As we have seen already, this allows many the potential to gain at least some independence in life, to find employment, and to obtain a degree of satisfaction and contentment.

This is a time when parents should be able to expect great sensitivity and good counselling skills on the part of doctors and others in attendance. If curative surgery is to be undertaken, they need good information presented in a simple and readily understandable way on the future prospect of their child. They also need guidance on the reasons behind the feelings they are experiencing; through insight of this kind they can begin to support each other. As a last resort doctors may turn to the law so that the child can be made a ward of court to minimise any delay of the curative surgery.

Unfortunately, the model of good practice outlined above has not always been apparent. Doctors' attitudes have been studied by David Silverman, working in a British paediatric cardiology clinic in the early 1980s. Using only a small sample, he highlighted a number of revealing issues. For example, in 10 consultations with parents of children with Down's syndrome, on not one occasion did the cardiologist ask 'Is he/she well?' In the 22 control families, 11 were greeted with this question. The inference here is that the physician made the assumption that a child with Down's syndrome could not be well and therefore did not bother to ask. It was also noted that, when the statement of diagnosis was made, in 75 per cent of the control families the anatomical description of the heart defect was tempered with some statement of reassurance.

Acknowledging that the heart defects in Down's syndrome might have been relatively more severe, it is noteworthy that in only one of 12 families studied at the diagnostic stage was there any such supportive statement. In the words of Silverman, many doctors seem to perceive that 'a child who is not altogether whole or is imperfect may turn out to be imperfectable'. In other words, the misunderstandings some doctors have about Down's syndrome may influence them when they are thinking about treatment, and some children may not get the treatment they deserve.

Doctors may also tend to discuss illnesses or problems identified by parents as 'just Down's syndrome' or 'typically Down's syndrome'. If not pursued, the lack of further investigation or follow-up can have serious consequences for development or health.

Previous authors have shown that medical judgment about mental ability in children with Down's syndrome made doctors predisposed not to intervene in congenital heart disease unless parents were actively in favour; for example, they were much more likely to operate upon a given heart condition where the child had a urogenital anomaly as opposed to Down's syndrome. Such prejudgement also exists in other areas. Doctors visiting families at home to decide on entitlement to attendance allowance the forerunner of Disability Living Allowance often assured the family of success (because their child had Down's syndrome) before any assessment of the child involved had actually taken place. Medical practitioners should not mix in their minds the concepts of health and handicap.

Reference has already been made to SCOPE's 'Right from the Start' campaign (page 37). It is hoped that as the medical and nursing professions learn more about how to introduce families to the idea that their child has a learning disability, doctors and nurses themselves will learn more of how to influence society to lessen the disadvantage of the condition.

Specific therapies for Down's syndrome

Pseudo-scientific vitamin regimes and intensive developmental programmes share a number of things in common. They are often presented to parents along with a grain of scientific truth, leading them to believe that they might actually represent a rational approach to therapy. The ideas that a vitamin concoction can radically alter body chemistry and that intensive stimulation can make brain cells grow both, on the face of it, seem tenable to the lay person. If one adds to this the ingredients of desperation, gullibility and a magical belief in the healing powers of health care professionals, then it is clear to see why some parents follow this course of action. Even though they may be told that scientific studies fail to show any benefit for the methods they are pursuing, they continue to pursue them because they want to feel they are doing something.

Meanwhile parents will find a variety of practitioners willing to advocate treatment of unproven value, often at some expense. Those involved are very vulnerable to this sort of suggestion. They may not have fully accepted their child's disability and yearn to put the problem right. Feelings of guilt may lead them to pursue any opportunity, no matter how spurious the treatment being offered. There is a whole series of treatments from centres throughout the world propounded by a very small number of medical practitioners, paramedical practitioners, hypnotists, allergists, cranial osteopaths, reflexologists and cell therapists, whose claims are at best intellectually dishonest, and possibly fraudulent.

Turkel advocates megavitamins for Down's syndrome, and there have been a number of exponents of this view. The approach is illogical because children with Down's syndrome have an increased gene dosage effect and vitamins only succeed by acting as co-enzymes, thus driving deficient rather than over-efficient enzyme systems. Long-term toxic effects of some vitamins, notably pyridoxine, vitamin B6, which causes a neuropathy, are documented. Where carefully controlled trials have been carried out, no benefit for this therapy has ever been shown.

Pauling was involved in some of the early studies of what has become known as orthomolecular medicine. He defined this as the treatment 'of mental disorders by the provision of the optimum molecular environment for the mind, especially the optimum concentration of substances normally present in the human body'. In the world of Down's syndrome, Harrell and colleagues (1981) published data on Turkel's 'U' series in

1964, indicating that vitamins enhanced the development of people with Down's syndrome. It must be said, though, that the choice of controls was poor and the work has proved to be unrepeatable.

Bennett and colleagues from Seattle (1983) carried out a randomised control trial of vitamin therapy versus placebo in 20 children with Down's syndrome aged between five and 13 years. The study subjects were matched for age, sex, race and socio-economic status. Over the eight-month period of the study no differences in the tested areas were found for development, behaviour, IQ, school achievement, speech and language or neuromotor function. Appearance, growth and health were also the same for the two groups. In the same year Smith and colleagues from Chicago, again using megadoses of vitamins, did a double-blind trial on 45 school-age children, again well matched for controls for measured intelligence, sex, age, and home and school environmental characteristics. They were assessed at baseline and after four and eight months, but no differences were seen on the measured variables.

Corman and colleagues carried out a double-blind study of vitamin B6 in infants with Down's syndrome. The rationale for their study resulted from an earlier observation that children with Down's syndrome had a significantly low level of 5-hydroxy-tryptamine (5HT). Administration of 5HT had led to the development of infantile spasms in one in six children so treated. Vitamin B6 is a co-enzyme in the second step of 5HT metabolism. Included in the complex is pyridoxal-5-phosphate, which is a major metabolite involved in the metabolism of brain amino acids, lipid nucleic acids and glycogen metabolism. It is mooted that the reduction in phospholipid content of myelin in Down's syndrome may be due to a relative deficiency of B6. The double-blind part of the study involved 19 infants of less than eight weeks of age. The treated group responded by having significantly elevated levels of 5HT, but this was only sustained during the first year of life. Growth rates, including head circumference, were exactly the same in the two groups at two years, as was all psychological testing. However, at six years the treated group had a significantly higher social quotient. This aspect of the work has not been repeated. In the open part of the study, where additional people with Down's syndrome were given

B6, a number of participants developed significant unwanted effects, blistering on exposure to sun, vomiting and the emergence of peripheral neuropathy being among the more serious. The peripheral neuropathy, well reported in other contexts, emerged after about four years' treatment. This illustrates well how the assumption cannot be that vitamins can do no harm. Any therapy used in Down's syndrome stands an equal chance of doing harm as possibly doing some good. Bumbalo and colleagues (1964) and Rowland and Spiker (1985) also failed to show benefit utilising double-blind procedures for nutritional treatment in Down's syndrome.

Advocates of so-called neurotransmitter therapy fail to acknowledge that the substances are probably not absorbed in their original form, and are therefore pharmacologically useless. Deanol (2-dimethylaminoethanol) is the substance usually mentioned by advocates of 'neurotransmitter therapy'. Deanol may be a precursor of acetylcholine; it has been claimed to enhance cholinergic activity. However, to claim this as its mode of action is purely speculative. The drug has been used in behaviour disorders and has been shown to improve performance in behaviourally disturbed children. Its effect is probably as a central stimulant, much the same as methylphenidate (Ritalin). These drugs carry the disadvantage that they may be addictive and can induce seizures. Ritalin might be considered very rarely for a child with Down's syndrome who has a particularly poor attention span and uncontrollable hyperactivity. Specialist advice is needed, and the drug is probably best used in a double-blind way alongside a placebo so that a good opinion may be formed on whether it is actually helping or not.

Cell therapy, equally, carries no logical rationale. Cell therapy originated in Europe and involves the injection of dried animal foetal cells on a five- to six-monthly basis. This is, however, rarely done in isolation, and advocates of the therapy usually combine it with a number of pharmacological preparations including vitamins, minerals and substances to treat the thyroid. Randomised double-blind controlled trials are difficult to carry out in these circumstances, where procedures are controversial, intrusive or potentially dangerous, but Foreman and Ward, working at Macquarie University, New South Wales, in Australia, have bravely tried. They compared two groups, one receiving and one not receiving cell therapy plus its associated medication. They placed a newsletter in the National Cell Therapy Association's magazine in Australia, and by this means identified 57 families receiving the therapy, of whom 53 were studied. Controls were matched for age and sex. No differences were found between the two groups in relation to growth and physical appearance (including skin and hair), nor on developmental quotients, save for the performance subscale of the Griffiths developmental scale for older children. The observed differences were significant but unimportant and, due to the study design, could well have been determined by confounding variables rather than treatment differences. Their study serves to show that where study groups are small the play of chance may serve to exaggerate or even underestimate the differences between groups. For example, taking the younger children as a whole on the performance scale, the mean score for treated children was 63.9 (SD 14.8) whereas that for controls was 77.1 (SD 16.3). This difference is not significant at the 5 per cent level. However, for older children the performance score for treated children was 57.5 (SD 13.0), whereas that for controls was 46.9 (SD 12.1). This difference is significant at the 5 per cent level but the effect is in the opposite direction to that seen in the younger child. Rather than the treatment having any real effect, a more likely conclusion is that chance has intervened to produce what is likely to be an unrepeatable result.

Piracetum is a drug that has received attention in recent years. In a controlled trial it was shown to improve the performance of children with specific learning difficulties. The advantage noted in the study was significant, measurable but in the classroom setting, arguably anyway, not all that important. The study has not been repeated and substantiated. It is, therefore, premature to suggest that the drug would be of benefit to young people with Down's syndrome. Further studies are required.

Facial plastic surgery

Since the early 1970s facial plastic surgery has been performed on many children with Down's syndrome, with the hope of 'normalising' the child's appearance, thus leading to better acceptance by society. Further objectives are to reduce drooling, facilitate better chewing and swallowing, and reduce the frequency of upper respiratory infections. Claims for the improvement of language development, cognitive function, social development and integration are also made. It must be noted, however, that 90 per cent of children with Down's syndrome do not drool, 85 per cent do not have significant difficulties with eating or chewing and three-quarters of parents feel that their child's facial features do not affect their social development in any negative way.

Partial glossectomy (removal of part of the tongue), lateral canthoplasty (refashioning the shape of the eyes) and enhancement of the zygoma (cheek bone) have all been advocated and carried out. Infection, the wound breaking down and foreshortening of the tongue have all been reported as complications, and time spent in hospital can unsettle children. Controlled assessment of the procedures has failed to show any overall benefit in appearance or articulatory ability.

It must be acknowledged that there may be pressing indications for plastic surgery in a very small number of children with Down's syndrome. Meanwhile, it would seem equally important to pay attention to appearance, dress sense and general hygiene so that acceptance by the child's peer group is more readily achieved.

Early intervention/intensive stimulation

Early intervention programmes are based on the premise that significant improvement in long-term developmental outcome can be achieved by ordered stimulation. Some have made claims that the stimulation actually leads to an increase in nerve cells. This claim is unsubstantiated, but there is animal work that infers that the developing brain hemispheres may retain a degree of plasticity if exposed to new stimuli. What is well established is that intervention programmes can help by offering psychological and social support to the families involved. Through help with adjustment, an environment is created in which opportunity and encouragement help children to reach their full potential.

There have been relatively few scientific evaluations of the benefit of intervention programmes. Studies have shown conflicting results, with benefit shown in some and none in others.

Ludlow and Allen studied home-reared children who did, or did not, receive an intervention programme and compared them with institutionalised children. The children on the intervention programme did best of all, with significantly less decline in developmental quotient beyond the age of three, and better performance following school entry. This was not, however, a randomised trial, and controls were not matched. In any study comparing developmental outcome it is essential to take note of variables such as number of siblings, socio-economic status and educational level of parents, as these are known to have a strong bearing on developmental attainment.

The work of Cunningham and Sloper is particularly to be commended in this regard. In one study they looked at 24 children at the age of 42 weeks, comparing those who received intensive training with a control group. The intensive training group received coaching on object performance, imitation and span of attention for one hour daily. The control group just got general advice. They found there were positive short-term effects for the intensive training group, but this good effect was not sustained. The intensive training group were able in the short term to improve performance in specific tasks.

In any learning process there is a period when the learning process reaches a plateau while the child consolidates the achievement. During this period the child may be unreliable in repeatedly performing the task, and his learned performance appears to be unstable. For example, during potty training a child may have occasional 'accidents' for quite a while before becoming reliably dry.

Cunningham and Sloper showed in their study that the short-term benefit was due to improved stability of performance. There was, however, no evidence that the intensive training was actually altering the processes by which the task was learnt, or that it was accelerating development by reducing the effects of cumulative disability. If they had noticed gains in these latter two respects, longer-term benefit might have been expected.

Their work also showed that there is a positive correlation between the mother's secondary educational achievement and developmental attainment in the child with Down's syndrome, implying that genetic, as well as psychosocial, factors operate to determine outcome. Children with Down's syndrome also did better when they had families who loved and valued them for who they were.

Nowadays a lot of pressure is put on parents, either from their own emotions or from the misguided energies of families or friends, to pursue intensive intervention programmes. The Doman Delacarto method is probably the best known, but it is just one of many. The American Academy of Pediatrics expressed concern over the Doman Delacarto programme in 1982. They found that the promotional methods often made it difficult for parents to refuse treatment; that the methods themselves were demanding, inflexible and stressful; that procedures put restrictions on age appropriate activities; and that, further, claims for dramatic improvement and cure were unsubstantiated. They commented that the treatment had no special merit, its claims were unproven and that the demands on families were so great that harm could result from its use.

Great caution certainly must be exercised before pursuing an intensive training programme, as the child's disability may well become the focus and *raison d'être* for all the family, to the detriment of any brothers and sisters. When disability within a family assumes this importance it really has become a handicap.

The driving forces for families coerced in this way are very complex, but non-acceptance of the disability and unresolved grief are clearly important in some. Where non-acceptance does persist, and parents retain an urge to 'put their child right', then they must be helped to realise that intensive training and pseudo-scientific dietary regimens will not alter the end result. Money raised for expensive trips to an institute for human potential or for exotic vitamin concoctions might more usefully be donated to local services, which are so often in need of extra resources.

There is no doubt that parents may turn to alternative therapy if they perceive the professionals they have to deal with are taking a negative attitude. Doctors, in particular, are all too readily accused of shaking their heads where disability is concerned (see pages 121–3). Equally, though, doctors and therapists must not fall into the trap of encouraging parents to believe they are 'healing'. There is a very fine line between presenting a therapy as something that will allow a person with Down's syndrome to develop their full potential and implying that the therapy will actually increase that potential to the point of cure. It is the magical belief that parents have in the healing powers of health professionals that take them off to institutes of therapy when they find themselves unable to adjust to the child's inherent rate of progress.

Community learning disability support

Most Primary Care Trusts now have a community learning disability support team who are in a position to advise parents on various aspects of their child's life, and this will be the mainstay of 'therapy'. A child with Down's syndrome spends most hours of the week at home with parents. Where the parents are well adjusted to the problem and where the child is loved and valued, the quality of interaction between parents and the child will be good too. It is therefore the aim of therapists to offer advice on the sort of interaction that might be pursued to encourage the next developmental step.

Most district health authorities will have a disability register so that facilities for individual children can be coordinated. Access to facilities can be obtained by general practitioner referral to a local paediatrician or senior clinical medical officer (local community clinic doctor). The diagnostic services available at the local district general hospital will help define any medical problems, and specialist advice will complement the original counselling process.

Physio- and occupational therapy

Much early development is dependent on motor skills. Children with Down's syndrome often have hypotonia (poor muscle tone), with poor muscle fixation at the shoulder and pelvis. Therapists can advise on the most suitable positioning, seating and play to develop these skills.

Speech therapy

Children with Down's syndrome often show language impairment over and above their general developmental disability. Initially, speech therapists can offer useful advice on the more severe speech problems, often in conjunction with the physiotherapist. Development of language concepts can be facilitated by the use of an alternative method of communication, such as Makaton, before speech develops. Some children with Down's syndrome reach school before speech has developed, but expressive language often improves at the same time as the acquisition of reading skills.

Speech therapy is a rare commodity in many local authorities. Nonetheless, parents should have confidence in themselves as teachers. What they do intuitively is often right!

Community nurse

The community nurse complements other members of the team by offering additional counselling, coordinating team members, giving out information and providing useful feedback. She may help families by introducing them to developmental checklists. Parents quickly forget what children learn to do in what order, and a rough guide on what comes next in any area of development, along with advice about what to include in play to facilitate this, may be welcome. There are many ways of achieving this. The approach may be unstructured or quite well defined, as in the Portage scheme, where parents keep a continuing record of progress.

Educational and clinical psychologists

At some stage a more formal assessment of developmental attainment will be appropriate, undertaken by an educational psychologist. The purpose of this is two-fold; the planning of education, and the counselling of parents. Assessments allow members of the team to counsel parents on the range of ability their child is likely to have in future years, and from the age of 10 months or so assessments take on a predictive quality in this respect; from this age counsellors can say with at least 80 per cent certainty that a child will be mildly, moderately or severely learning impaired. Care must be taken not to confuse intellectual with social ability, remembering it is possible to be illiterate but to be quite able to care for oneself.

The psychologist is usually the best local person to provide parents with information on schools. The 1981 Education Act states that children with special needs are entitled to the benefits of education from the age of two, although it must be acknowledged that not all education authorities have the resources to meet all children's needs. Usually, however, a good compromise can be reached between a family's hopes and expectations and what is actually available. Medical practitioners are asked to contribute to statements of special educational need, and that evidence is considered along with formal and semi-formal educational assessments (see Chapter 7). Very often it will be obvious where the child is best placed in school; at other times a trial placement must be made.

Clinical psychologists can offer useful child guidance if behavioural problems are causing stress within the family. The key aims are to help families identify the source of the child's frustration, and hopefully to overcome it. Consistency in approach is very important, not only between family members but with staff at school, too.

At times behaviour patterns are more determined by the underlying brain problem itself rather than by the child's environment, particularly in the more severely disabled. In these circumstances behavioural therapy will not be wholly successful, and parents should be encouraged to seek respite care through local social services, and especially to do it without any feeling of shame or failure.

Social services and benefits

Although limited resources may not allow the provision of a social worker for every community learning disability team, families are advised to have at least one consultation with the local department of social services.

Social services should also be asked what provision they are making for the care of the adult disabled within their authority. There are two aspects to this:

- What plans for provision have actually been made?
- Is funding available?

Generally, good special educational facilities exist within authorities, but once children leave school, arrangements are far less satisfactory. Parents should be encouraged to press local authorities to draw up plans for such provision where they do not exist.

Meanwhile social workers can be very helpful in arranging respite care where it is needed. In childhood and teenage years this is often on a short-term basis initially. Local authorities have a number of small community homes for this purpose, but are increasingly recruiting families in the community to act as foster parents and to offer the children a 'home from home'. Parents are bound to feel reticent about this initially, although it is surprising how children often relish the experience of 'weekends away'. The foster parents usually have children of their own, and it turns out to be something of an adventure for all concerned.

During school holidays Social services often run play-schemes for the learning-disabled.

For advice on benefits we recommend going to a welfare benefits advice agency, such as the Welfare Rights Unit (run by local authorities), a CAB, a local Disability Information Advice Line (DIAL), a local MENCAP office, or contacting the welfare benefits advisers at the DSA.

Benefits that people with Down's syndrome and their families may be entitled to include:

- **Disability Living Allowance** This benefit is to compensate for the extra costs of having a disability. It is not means-tested. It has two parts – a 'care component' and a 'mobility component'. The care component can be claimed from when a child is three months old. It is given for children who need a lot more help with personal care than other children of the same age. 'Personal care' is help with dressing, washing, eating, drinking, going to the toilet, sleeping, crawling, walking, speaking, hearing, playing, etc. It includes help with encouraging and prompting a child with Down's syndrome to learn. 'Personal care' also includes the need for extra supervision. All children with Down's syndrome should get this benefit, though it can be difficult deciding when to apply.

  The higher rate of the mobility component can be claimed when a child is three years old if they are having problems learning to walk or if they have serious behavioural difficulties. Otherwise, the lower rate can be claimed at the age of five. Again, everyone with Down's syndrome should qualify for at least the lower rate of the mobility component.

- **Carer's Allowance** This is for people who are not working because they are looking after someone with an illness or disability. If you are not working (or only earning a small amount) and your child is receiving DLA (at the middle or higher rate of the care component), then you may get the Carer's Allowance.
- **Working Tax Credit** This will help disabled people who are working but whose income is not high.
- **Means-tested benefits** Means-tested benefits include Job-seeker's Allowance, Income Support, Housing Benefit, Council Tax Benefit, Child Tax Credit and Working Tax Credit. Having a child with a disability (that is, a child who gets DLA) may mean that you get higher amounts of the means-tested benefits.

The benefits system is complicated. This is only a very brief summary. It is a good idea to get advice from a specialist welfare benefits adviser on your own situation. It is especially important to get advice when claiming Disability Living Allowance.

Summary

There is no evidence to suggest that either intensive intervention programmes or nutritional treatment alter the developmental potential of people with Down's syndrome in any important way. Parents often turn to these methods where they have found negative attitudes amongst the professionals they deal with or where they have unresolved grief and non-acceptance of the disability. Changing the attitudes of doctors will take time, but unresolved parental grief and non-acceptance of the disability can both be helped with counselling.

Children with Down's syndrome spend most hours of the week at home with their parents. Where the parents are well adjusted to the problem and where the child is loved and valued, the quality of interaction between parents and child will be naturally good. It should then be the aim of therapists to offer advice on the sort of interaction that is most likely to encourage the next developmental step.

Children with Down's syndrome are likely to do best where they are loved and valued for the individuals they are, and when they have good local professional advice to complement the loving encouragement of their parents.

11

Growing up with Down's syndrome in the 21st century

The human genome project

Begun formally in 1990, the Human Genome Project is coordinated by the U.S. Department of Energy and the National Institutes of Health. The project was originally planned to last 15 years, but rapid technological advances have accelerated the expected completion date to 2003. The project's aims are to:

- identify all the approximate 30,000 genes in human DNA;
- determine the sequences of the three billion chemical base pairs that make up human DNA;
- store this information in databases;
- improve tools for data analysis;
- transfer related technologies to the private sector;
- address the ethical, legal and social issues (ELSI) that may arise from the project – the first large scientific project to do so.

The practical benefits of learning about DNA include the possibility of discovering revolutionary new ways to diagnose, treat and someday prevent the thousands of disorders that affect the human population. In May 2000 scientists identified all the genes located on chromosome 21. Continuing research will identify which genes on chromosome 21 are responsible for the more disabling characteristics associated with Down's syndrome, such as learning disability, congenital cardiac defects, immunological deficiencies and Alzheimer's disease. This may lead to devising treatments and/or therapies to improve the health and wellbeing of people with Down's syndrome. How far-reaching these treatments may be is not at all clear at this stage. It is important, though, that the research initiatives and legislation governing genetic testing and gene therapies continue to reflect the dignity, worth and equal rights of all people, regardless of mental and physical capacity.

The prospects are exciting. We may learn, too, more about why having Down's syndrome is in some instances a health advantage: why there are very low rates of arteriosclerosis (hardening of the arteries), and many solid tumours (a type of cancer) and why multiple sclerosis is almost unknown.

Therapy?

Probably the best therapy any child – or adult for that matter – can have is love, opportunity and encouragement. There is no convincing evidence that intensive therapy of any sort (physical, occupational or educational) will allow children to learn any faster than they are able. The brain is so very eager to learn that when it is ready it will learn. This is an important message for parents, as it takes the pressure off and allows them to feel they are doing enough. As our educational system for integration and inclusion improves, the future is for parents, classroom helpers and teachers to work together to offer that opportunity and encouragement.

One young man with Down's syndrome recently left secondary school to go on to sixth form college. Off his own bat he asked to address the school at the leavers' assembly. He took to the stage timidly and spoke. The 300 assembled pupils treated him with respect as they awaited what he had to say; you could have heard a pin drop. 'Thank you for helping me and being my friend,' he said. That was all, but the hall erupted into cacophonous, generous and genuine applause. There was a tear in the eye of assembled parents, teachers and helpers. They had witnessed over the years from primary through secondary education an initial acknowledgement of difference and then a growth of mutual respect between the boy with Down's syndrome and others (of similar ability in many respects) within the school and the peer group. They did not think it uncool to be seen with him, enjoyed singing and dancing together at the leavers' ball, shouted hello across the street in town and welcomed social outings. An education system that includes will produce new generations of people who will include rather than marginalise, and will recognise the worthiness of all people.

Meanwhile, the temptation is still there to try this drug and that vitamin to boost performance. It must be remembered, however, that there is no substance on earth that can do good without the capacity to do harm. All drugs, including enzymes and co-enzymes, have unwanted as well as wanted effects. Usually, but not always, the wanted effects are seen first. As we learn more about the biochemistry of Down's syndrome we should expect to see new rational treatment options appear. The only ethical way to introduce them is by means of structured research programmes under the proper direction of qualified people so that the wanted and unwanted effects of the intervention can be monitored as they become known. In this way safe remedies will emerge and our knowledge will grow.

Social policy, legislation and education

Whereas it is plain to see that huge advances in all sorts of areas have taken place since Langdon Down recognised but one form of learning disability in the 1860s, there remains very much more to be achieved. Enormous change in social policy and legislation has taken place, especially over the last 50 years, which has directly affected the lives of people with Down's syndrome and their families. Two of the biggest changes have been the right to education and an end to institutional care in long-stay hospitals.

A right to education was denied until 1971. More recently people have been entitled legally to the right to an education in a school of their own choosing, which has led to more and more children with Down's syndrome attending mainstream school. We are also now beginning to see adults with Down's syndrome who have attended mainstream school right the way from primary through secondary school. This generation, as we have seen, are leaving school with the same hopes and aspirations as their peers – to leave home, find a job and form a relationship; however, these are much harder to realise for adults with Down's syndrome, largely due to the lack of financial support and access to appropriate services to make these dreams a reality.

The closure of the long-stay hospitals has also brought about significant change in people's lives. Many such hospitals were dumping grounds where there was little education and certainly very little health care, ironic for hospital settings. At the same time, although thousands of people were incarcerated in these institutions, most children and adults actually remained at home with their families and with no official community support. The closure of these places and the recognition that people with learning disabilities could lead ordinary lives within their communities became enshrined in community care legislation, which offered financial support and access to appropriate services for *the individual*.

However, the reality of this was that many people with Down's syndrome were not receiving appropriate support and again were being denied the right to live lives of their own choosing. The Government recognised this and recently completed the first full review of services for people with learning disabilities in 30 years. This has resulted in the White Paper 'Valuing People: A New Strategy for Learning Disability in the 21st Century'. The key principles, perhaps philosophy, in this White Paper are that legal and civil rights, independence, choice, and inclusion are to be reflected in every aspect of the lives of children and adults with learning disabilities. (This White Paper applies only to England, though similar strategies are being introduced in Scotland, Wales and Northern Ireland.)

Person Centred Planning is one of the key instruments in making this happen. Person Centred Planning means looking at the individual and what rights and choices they have in their life. People with Down's syndrome are as individual in their likes and dislikes as the rest of the population, but they are often not listened to or facilitated in communication so that they can let their preferences be known. For many years the diagnostic label, and the stereotype attached to this, has determined the lives that people have been left to lead:

Down's syndrome = group home, horticultural training course, group day out?

This diagnostic labelling does not take into account that A, an adult with Down's syndrome, does not choose to live with seven other people in a group home, hates gardening and loathes the day out on the special minibus to the seaside. A has other interests. However, that is also not to say that B, an adult with Down's syndrome, does not love living with seven other people, and adore gardening, and could not think of a better day out than the special minibus trip to the seaside. B has preferences, too. There is the real danger in service provision that a forward-thinking philosophy and culture is embraced with such well-meaning ferocity that, once again, the rights and choices of people with Down's syndrome are denied.

In order to help people with Down's syndrome to make their hopes and aspirations become a reality we all must strive for them to achieve equality – to live in a society in which they are as valued and have the same human and civil rights as everyone else. We also must not lose sight of their individuality and right to live a life of their own choosing.

A quote from a man with Down's syndrome who has bought his own home and is living by himself with support captures this:

'Soup for breakfast, now that is what I call independence!'

[illegible]

[illegible] an increment to remove [illegible] are [illegible] found in the [illegible] [illegible]

[illegible] produced by [illegible] the [illegible] and the [illegible] [illegible] larger than average [illegible]

chalazion [illegible] an inflammation present in the [illegible] A [illegible] of [illegible] which [illegible] at a [illegible] [illegible]

[illegible] [illegible] of [illegible] [illegible] [illegible] to an [illegible] [illegible] [illegible] produced by the [illegible] which [illegible] and [illegible]

[illegible] A drug that boosts the [illegible] by preventing [illegible] Chemical substances such as vitamin [illegible] which [illegible] oxidative processes [illegible] and [illegible] the production of damaging [illegible] an abnormality of the eye [illegible] vision in more than one place.

[illegible] of the [illegible] [illegible] with advancing [illegible] the [illegible] [illegible] [illegible] the [illegible]

GLOSSARY

Adenoidectomy An operation to remove the adenoids, which are lymph glands found in the upper part of the throat known as the naso-pharynx.

Alopecia Areas of baldness.

Alpha-fetoprotein Protein produced by the foetal liver which passes into the amniotic fluid and the maternal circulation, where it is found in increased amounts in some foetal abnormalities or in lower than average amounts in Down's syndrome.

Alphatocopherol An antioxidant present in the diet.

Alzheimer's Disease A cause of pre-senile dementia (in which people lose their faculties at an early age) which is common in Down's syndrome.

Amniocentesis The drawing off of some amniotic fluid contained in the sac which surrounds the growing foetus.

Amyloid A protein coded for on chromosome 21.

Aneuploidy Too many or too few chromosomes.

Anterior commissure Connecting fibres between the two frontal lobes of the brain.

Antibodies Proteins produced by the body's immune system which help to neutralise infecting agents such as bacteria or viruses.

Anticholinesterase A drug that boosts the level of a neuro-transmitter called acetylcholine by preventing its breakdown.

Antioxidant Chemical substances such as vitamin E or alpha-tocopherol which inhibit oxidative processes in cells and thereby reduce the production of damaging free radicals.

Astigmatism An abnormality of the eye lens which distorts vision in more than one plane.

Atheroma A type of degeneration of the walls of arteries (main blood vessels) seen with advancing age.

Atlanto-axial instability The tendency for the first cervical vertebrum (the atlas) to slip on the second (the axis).

Atresia Failure in development of the hole through a hollow organ such as a bowel or blood vessel.

Atrium One of two low pressure chambers of the heart receiving blood from veins to pass on to the ventricles.

Autoantibodies Proteins produced by the body's immune system which have the potential to damage the body's own tissue.

Autoimmune disease A disorder of a variety of organs, caused by the production of autoantibodies.

Beta-blockers Drugs that prevent the heart from being raced by the excitatory autonomic nervous system.

Biofeedback Mechanisms that control body functions with the use of sensors or receptors which are sensitive to the level of specific chemicals (and therefore switch off production for a while) or the level of nervous impulses, as seen in the control of muscle tone.

Brainstem The long thin part of the brain on which the cerebral hemisphere and cerebellum lie. It contains the control centres for the muscles of the head and neck and vital bodily functions such as breathing.

Brushfield spots Speckling of the iris.

Canalisation Direction and organisation of a developmental process such as organ formation.

Cataract Opaque deposits in the eye lens causing difficulty with vision.

Cell A small discrete mass from which most living things are made, containing the protoplasm in which most of the chemical reactions on which life is dependent take place bounded by the cell-wall; in the centre is a nucleus containing the chromosomal material that directs the chemical processes.

Central nervous system The brain and spinal cord.

Centromere The spindle attachment of chromosomes.

Cerebellum One of the main motor control centres of the brain which receives and coordinates sensory information to modify motor output.

Chiasmata Connections between chromatids, visible during meiosis.

Chorionic villus biopsy Sampling of tissue from the sac containing the developing foetus, usually at about 12 weeks of gestational age.

Chromosome Thread-shaped body of which there are normally 23 pairs in the nucleus of each cell; made largely of DNA, they govern cell structure and function.

Chromatid One of two strands of a chromosome formed when the DNA material duplicates during mitosis or meiosis.

Coeliac disease Disease of the intestine leading to the malabsorption of nutrients, due to sensitivity to the gluten contained in cereals.

Coenzyme A substance, often a vitamin, playing an essential part in the reactions of enzyme systems; it avoids being consumed in the process because it is used in one step of the reaction but reconstituted by a later step.

Cranial nerve Peripheral nerve emerging from the brain to supply structures of the head.

Cutis marmorata Mottled skin rash taking up the pattern of the underlying small blood vessels.

Cyanosis Blueness of the tissues due either to poor blood supply or low oxygen concentration in the blood.

Cyclid guanine monophosphate The specific substance or substrate acted on by the enzyme guanylate cyclase, generating energy for cell wall function.

Cystathionine synthase An enzyme involved in the production of cystathionine that seems to protect against arteriosclerosis.

Dendrites Branching projections of nerve-cells which pass on and receive impulses from neighbouring nerves.

Dentition Arrangement of the teeth.

Differentiation Process of change in groups of cells as they form the different tissues and organs of the body both during foetal development and after injury.

Digoxin Drug to slow and increase the strength of the heart beat.

Disability The relatively poor function that results from a physical impairment, such as the poor vision that might result from cataracts.

DNA Deoxyribonucleic acid, a large number of nucleotides linked with a parallel strand by base-pairs and coiled in a helix. It is found mainly in the chromosomes, where its power to reproduce some of the sequences of nucleotides leads to the production of proteins that make up cell structure and function.

DNA probe Chemical marker capable of identifying and locking on to a specific sequence of nucleotides.

Duodenum First part of the small intestine, leading from the stomach.

Dysembryogenesis Disorderly formation of an organ at an early stage in uterine life.

Dysfunction A disorder or malfunction.

Dyspraxia Difficulty in carrying out movements in a fluent way in spite of having a full capacity to move and with no weakness; poor coordination and sequencing of movement by the brain.

Dystrophic Disordered growth of an organ or system.

Echocardiography Imaging of the heart using ultra-sound.

Endocardial cushion A swelling of atrial canal tissue seen in the early embryo which acts as a seat for the mitral and tricuspid valves and from which the atrio-ventricular septum is formed.

Endocrine glands The glands that produce hormones.

Endoplasmic reticulum Complex system of paired membranes lying in the cytoplasm of the cell which contain many of the cell's enzyme systems.

Epicanthic folds The fold of skin seen at the inner nasal side of the eye.

Epilepsy A recurring abnormality of posture or tone, usually associated with an alteration of conscious level due to abnormal electrical discharge in the brain.

Folate Dietary substance that promotes normal growth in red blood and nerve-cells in particular.

Follicle-stimulating hormone Hormone produced by the pituitary gland which promotes the normal production of eggs and sperm.

Fore-brain The anterior, front division of the embyronic brain, from which are formed the cerebral hemispheres, eyes and part of the pituitary gland.

Free radical Oxygen-containing biochemical which can damage the energy production in cells if overproduced.

Gamete An egg or sperm.

Gene A unit of DNA on the chromosome which is responsible for the production of a specific protein.

Glossectomy Surgical removal of the tongue (usually partial).

Glutathione peroxidase An enzyme that helps to control the production of free radicals.

Glycogen A biochemical made up of many glucose molecules; the form in which glucose is stored, particularly in the muscles and liver.

Gonadotrophin The small group of hormones secreted by the pituitary gland that control the function of the ovaries and testicles.

Grommet Small, holed device which may be inserted into the ear-drum to effect drainage of fluid from the middle ear.

Guanylate-cyclase A membrane enzyme system that produces energy.

Handicap A disadvantage for an individual resulting from a disability and impairment which limits or prevents the fulfilment of a role or task. Poor coordination (the disability) due to brain structure (the impairment in Down's syndrome) may be a handicap when playing football but not when watching television.

Heteromorphism The variation of chromosomal structure which results from the crossing over of DNA from one to another at cell division.

Hyperextension Overextension.

Hyperkeratosis Scaliness of the skin due to an overproduction of keratin.

Hypermetropia Long-sightedness.

Hyperploidy More than the usual number of chromosomes.

Hyperthyroid The clinical state resulting from an overactive thyroid gland.

Hypoplasia Under-growth of an organ.

Hypoploidy Less than the usual number of chromosomes.

Hypospadias Where the urethral opening (the exit hole for urine) falls short of the tip of the penis.

Hypothalamus Part of the brain that governs the function of the pituitary gland and the autonomic (automatic) nervous system.

Hypothyroid Clinical state associated with an underactive thyroid gland.

Hypotonia Where the resting activity in muscles (tone) is lower than usual.

Immune system/Immunity The body's defence system,

partly effected by lymphocytes (small white blood cells) produced in the thymus gland and partly by antibodies produced by lymphocytes originating elsewhere in the lymphatic system.

Impairment An abnormality of structure of an organ which may lead to a disability.

Interferon A complex protein with anti-viral properties.

Lacrimal gland The gland that produces tears.

Lecithin Fatty substance made up of glycerol, fatty acid, choline and phosphoric acid found in animal cells.

Leukaemia Cancerous overproduction of white blood cells.

Limbic system Part of the brain which includes the hypothalamus; it controls the autonomic (automatic) nervous system, the interpretation of smell and some aspects of learning.

Lipoperoxidation The involvement of fatty acids and cholesterol in oxidative metabolism (the adding of oxygen to their structure) which may disrupt cell structure and function if not well controlled.

Luteinising hormone A gonadotrophin important in the control of ovulation.

Lymphocyte-functional antigen A substance that assists the binding of lymphocytes to foreign material (antigen).

Macroscopic Seen by the naked eye.

Makaton Simple system of sign language.

Malabsorption A deficiency in which food contents are taken into the circulation due to poor function of the bowel wall.

Meiosis Two successive cell divisions which resemble mitosis, but the chromosomes are only duplicated once, resulting in this being the reduction division.

Membrane A layer of molecules that form a barrier.

Metabolism The chemical processes involved in living organisms which build up (anabolism) or break down (catabolism) organic biochemicals.

Methotrexate An anti-folate chemical used in the treatment of leukaemia.

Microscopic Seen only down the microscope; too small to be seen with the naked eye.

Microtubules The tiny filaments that make up the spindles at cell division.

Mitosis The usual process of cell division: the chromosomes duplicate and then there is a separation of these duplicates so that each daughter cell has the normal number of chromosomes.

Monoclonal antibody An antibody produced by a single cell line (clone) very specifically for a single antigen.

Monocyte Largest white cell involved in clearing the products of inflammation.

Mosaicism Where the body is made up of more than one population of cells, one with the normal number of chromosomes and the other with an abnormal number of chromosomes.

Myelography Special X-ray examination designed to outline the spinal cord.

Myopia Short-sightedness.

Myringotomy Opening up of the ear-drum.

Nasolacrimal duct The tunnel through the tissues which joins the eye to the nose down which many tears pass.

Neuritic plaques One of the microscopic hallmarks of Alzheimer's disease seen in brain tissue.

Neurofibrillary tangles Another microscopic hallmark of Alzheimer's disease seen in brain tissue.

Neuropathy A disorder of the function of peripheral nerves, which take information from the brain out from the spinal cord to the muscles.

Neurotransmitter A chemical released from a nerve ending which crosses the synapse to excite or inhibit activity in the adjoining nerve-cell.

Non-disjunction Failure of two similar (homologous) chromosomes to go to opposite poles at the first meiotic division so that one daughter cell has both of the pair and one has neither.

Nucleic acid Long-chain molecule such as DNA made up of a large number of nucleotides.

Nucleus The part of the cell that contains the chromosomes.

Odontoid process/peg A bony projection of the second cervical vertebrum (axis) which passes into a hole in the body of the first cervical verberum (atlas), thus forming the pivot for rotation of the head on the neck.

Oestriol An oestrogen hormone whose concentration rises during pregnancy, when it is produced largely by the placenta.

Oncogene A cancer-susceptibility gene.

Ossicle One of the bones making up the sound-conducting mechanism in the middle ear.

Paroxysmal Of sudden onset.

Phenotype The characteristic appearance or manifestation of a particular genetic make-up (the genotype).

Phosphofructokinase An enzyme involved in the metabolism of glucose.

Polyhydramnios Where too much amniotic fluid surrounds the foetus.

Positron-emission tomography Three-dimensional imaging of the brain to display specific biochemical functions by using radio-active isotopes.

Primitive reflexes Involuntary, reflex patterns of movement seen in the developing foetus or young infant, usually controlled at spinal or brain-stem level, which disappear in the first few months of life as more complex patterns of movement emerge.

Proteinaceous Largely made up of protein.

Psychosis Disorder of the mind or mental illness which interferes with a person's ability to make sense of the world and what is seen, heard or felt.

Purines Biochemicals including adenine and guanine which are some of the base-building blocks that make up DNA.

Pyridoxal-5-phosphate Related to vitamin B6, this plays an important part in brain metabolism.

Pyrimidines Biochemicals including thymine and cytosine which are some of the base-building blocks that make up DNA.

Ritalin An addictive drug (other name methylphenidate) which has been used in the control of hyperactive behaviour.

Schilling test A test to evaluate the absorption of vitamin B12.

Seborrhoeic dermatatis An inflammatory, scaling condition of hairy areas of skin which have a lot of sebaceous glands.

Selenium A trace element essential for a number of enzyme systems.

Septum Partition or wall.

Serotonin Also known as 5-hydroxytryptamine, this is an important neurotransmitter.

Serum Blood plasma minus its clotting constituents.
Somatomedin An important growth hormone produced by the pituitary gland.
Spermatogenesis The normal process of sperm production by the testicle.
Spinal cord The part of the central nervous system that lies in the backbone; the nerve fibres are taking motor information down to and transmitting sensory information up from each segmental level of the body.
Spindle Body formed in cells during mitosis and meiosis which takes part in the distribution of the chromatids to the two daughter nuclei.
Standard deviation (SD) A statistical measure of the spread or variability of the probability distribution around the mean. A small standard deviation means the distribution is close to the mean. A large value indicates a wide range of possible outcomes.
Stenosis Abnormal narrowing of a hollow structure such as a blood vessel or bowel.
Superoxide dismutase Enzyme involved in the metabolism of binding oxygen to biochemicals; the result is the production of free radicals.
T cell Thymus-dependent lymphocytes involved in cell-mediated body defences.
Testosterone The principal male sex-steroid hormone.
Thymus gland A primary lymphoid organ in the upper part of the chest where T cells mature.
Thyroid An endocrine gland in the neck which produces hormones that control growth and the rate of body metabolism.
Thyroxine Hormone produced by the thyroid gland.
Trace element A substance that must be available to the body in very small amounts to ensure good health: trace elements act as constituents in enzyme systems e.g. copper, molybdenum, selenium and so on.
Translocation Transfer of part of a chromosome onto a different part of a chromosome of the same type (homologous) or a different (non-homologous) type.
Trial A method of working out the effectiveness of a treatment (a drug or perhaps a method of physiotherapy). The effect of the treatment is measured in a study group

and compared to a control group of subjects who had no treatment or perhaps a long-established method of treatment. Placebos are often used in the control group. Trials may be double-blind, where neither doctor nor subject know whether the treatment is drug or placebo (a record of treatment usually being kept by a third person such as a pharmacist).

Tri-iodothyronine A hormone produced by the thyroid gland.

Trimester One of three, three-month periods that make up pregnancy in humans.

Trisomy Describes a nucleus containing three of one type of chromosome instead of the usual two.

Tympanic membrane The ear-drum.

Tympanosclerosis Distortion of the ear-drum with scar-tissue.

Ventricle A chamber. There are two in the heart, which act as the muscular pumping chambers. There are four in the brain, through which and in which the cerebro-spinal fluid flows.

Vertibrum One of the bones making up the spinal column, through which passes the spinal cord.

Vitamins Substances that are vital for normal body metabolism, usually acting as co-enzymes ensuring the smooth and fast running of enzyme-systems.

Vitiligo Skin condition in which areas of the skin contain no pigment, at times associated with autoimmune disease elsewhere in the body.

Zygoma The cheek bone.

ABOUT THE DOWN'S SYNDROME ASSOCIATION AND ITS MISSION

The Down's Syndrome Association was founded in 1970 as the Down's Babies Association. It grew with its original families to become the Down's Children's Association in 1973, and finally the Down's Syndrome Association in 1986. The Down's Syndrome Association is now the main UK charitable organisation covering all aspects of living with Down's syndrome. Our driving ambition is to create the conditions that all people with Down's syndrome need in order to live lives of their own choosing.

- We provide information and support for people with Down's syndrome, and their families and carers, as well as being a resource for interested professionals.
- We work to improve knowledge and understanding of the condition amongst all our audiences, including the general public, government services and a wide range of interested groups.
- We champion the rights of people with Down's syndrome, campaigning for change and challenging discrimination.
- The DSA provides direct help to members in England, Wales and Northern Ireland, and others through:
  - our telephone helpline and advocacy services;
  - our wide range of publications, including accessible information for people with Down's syndrome;
  - our campaigning activities;
  - our Journal, with advice, articles and news and views;
  - our *Down 2 Earth* Magazine, written for and by adults with Down's syndrome.

USEFUL ADDRESSES

British Institute of Learning Disabilities
Campion House
Green Street
Kidderminster
Worcestershire DY10 1JL
Tel: 01562 723010
Fax: 01562 723029
www.bild.org.uk

The Down's Heart Group
National Family Support Coordinator
17 Cantilupe Close
Eaton Bray
Dunstable
Beds LU6 2EA
Tel: 01525 220379
www.downs-heart.downsnet.org

Down's Syndrome Educational Trust
Sarah Duffen Centre
Belmont Street
Southsea
Hants PO5 1NA
Tel: 02392 855300
www.downsed.org

Down's Syndrome Ireland
30 Mary Street
Dublin 1
Tel: 00 353 1 873 0999
Fax: 00 353 1 873 3612

Down's Syndrome Scotland
158–160 Balgreen Road
Edinburgh EH11 3AU
Tel: 0131 313 4225
www.dscotland.org.uk

Foundation for People with Learning Disabilities
83 Victoria Street
London SW1H OHW
Tel: 020 7802 0300
Fax: 020 7802 0301
www.learningdisabilities.org.uk

Mencap
123 Golden Lane
London EC1Y ORT
Tel: 020 7454 0454
Fax: 020 7696 5540
www.mencap.org.uk

VIA – Values into Action
Oxford House
Derbyshire Street
London E2 6HG
Tel: 020 7729 5436
Fax: 020 7729 7797
www.viauk.org

WEBSITES

DownsEd
Website for parents and professionals promoting education and development through research and information.
www.downsed.org

The Down's Syndrome Medical Interest Group (DSMIG)
DSMIG is a network of doctors from the UK and Republic of Ireland who have a special interest in Down's syndrome. Very useful site for medical information.
www.dsmig.org.uk

Independent Panel for Special Education Advice (IPSEA)
IPSEA offers free and independent advice on Local Education Authorities' legal duties to assess and provide for children with special educational needs.
www.ipsea.org.uk

Information for medical professionals and students
A website developed and managed by the Down's Syndrome Association in conjunction with St George's Hospital Medical School. This resource provides comprehensive information for health students and professionals on all aspects of caring for someone with Down's syndrome.
www.intellectualdisability.info/home.htm

Len Leshin
Medical advice on a wide range of subjects and links to international related sites.
www.ds-health.com

Mosaic Down's syndrome
Site for specific information on Mosaic Down's syndrome.
www.mosaicdownsyndrome.com

The Society for the Study of Behavioural Phenotypes
International organisation of doctors, psychologists and research workers set up to investigate behavioural and emotional aspects of biologically determined syndromes associated with intellectual disability.
www.ssbp.co.uk

UK People First Organisation
An organisation of people with learning difficulties speaking up for themselves. People First is run and controlled by people with learning difficulties.
www.peoplefirst.org.uk

UK resources for Down's syndrome
A comprehensive set of addresses and links for Down's syndrome in the UK on the web. Includes links to government agencies, voluntary organisations and the full text of the 1996 Education Act.
www.43green.freeserve.co.uk/uk_downs_syndrome/ukdsinfo.html

FURTHER READING

Adolescents with Down's Syndrome
S. M. Pueschel & M. Sustrova. Paul Brookes 1997

Down's Syndrome: A Review of Current Knowledge
Ed. by J. Rondal, J. Perera, L. Nadel. Whurr Publishers 1999

Down's Syndrome and Health Care
Vee Prasher & Beryl Smith, BILD Publications 2002

Down's Syndrome: The Facts
Mark Selikowitz. Oxford University Press 1997

The Down's Syndrome Nutrition Handbook: A Guide to Promoting Healthy Lifestyles
Joan Guthrie Medlen. Woodbine House 2002

Down's Syndrome: Visions for the 21st Century
Ed. by W. I. Cohen, L. Nadel, M. Madnick. Wiley-Liss 2002

Early Communication Skills for Children with Down's Syndrome: A Guide for Parents and Professionals
Libby Kumin. Woodbine House 2003

Fine Motor Skills in Children with Down's Syndrome: A Guide for Parents and Professionals
Maryanne Bruni, Woodbine House 1997

Gross Motor Skills in Children with Down's Syndrome: A Guide for Parents and Professionals
Patricia Winders. Woodbine House 1997

Medical & Surgical Care for Children with Down's Syndrome: A Guide for Parents
Ed. by D. C. Van Dyke & P. Mattheis. Woodbine House 1995

New Approaches to Down's Syndrome
Ed. by Brian Stratford & Pat Gunn. Cassell 1996

Teaching Reading to Children with Down's Syndrome: A Guide for Parents and Teachers
Patricia Oelwein. Woodbine House 1995

INDEX

Numbers in *italic* indicate illustrations.